Clinical
Handbook
Supportive
Care

Advanced Individual
Training Course
91W10

Clinical Handbook
Supportive Care

Advanced Individual Training Course

91W10

Clinical Handbook Supportive Care: Advanced Individual
Training Course 91W10

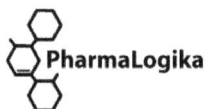

PharmaLogika

PharmaLogika, Inc.
PO Box 461
Willow Springs, NC 27592

www.pharmalogika.com

PharmaLogika Books is an imprint of PharmaLogika, Inc.
PharmaLogika and its logos are trademarks of PharmaLogika, Inc.
All other trademarks used herein are the properties of their
respective owners and are used for identification purposes only.

Author / Editor: Mindy J. Allport-Settle

Published by PharmaLogika, Inc.

Printed in the United States of America.

ISBN 0-9830719-7-7
ISBN-13 978-0-9830719-7-6

Contents

Supportive Care 2

Supportive Care 3

Supportive Care 4

Overview

About this Book

The United States Army is recognized internationally as the standard for complete, efficient and effective adult education. The Army has a tradition of pioneering training systems (including computer-based training) that then transition into the corporate sector. This manual has been continuously tested and updated to successfully educate every member of the modern United States Army. The needs of the instructor, the student, and the Army are perfectly balanced. This is the model all educators strive to follow when developing and delivering training programs.

Included Documents and Features

Supportive Care 1

- Treat Metabolic Endocrine Symptoms
- Treat Neurological Symptoms
- Treat Cardiopulmonary Symptoms
- Treat Gastrointestinal Symptoms
- Treat Genitourinary Symptoms
- Treat Skin Disorders
- Treat infectious Disease & Immunologic Symptoms
- Competency Skill Sheets

Supportive Care 2

- Manage a Seizing Casualty

- Assist in Vaginal Delivery
- Perform Medical Screening
- Immunization and Chemoprophylaxis
- Specimen Collection
- Blood Draw
- Competency Skill Sheets

Supportive Care 3

- Basic Nursing Assessment
- Nursing Documentation
- Medication Administration
- Pain Assessment and Management
- Pharmacology for the Soldier Medic

Supportive Care 4

- Post-Mortem Care
- Wound Care
- Perform Respiratory Care
- Cardiac Monitoring
- Chest Tube Care and Monitoring
- Competency Skill Sheets

Orientation

Health Care Ethics

Health care ethics (also known as *medical ethics*) is a system of moral principles that apply values and judgments to the practice of medicine. As a scholarly discipline, medical ethics encompasses its practical application in clinical settings as well as work on its history, philosophy, theology, and sociology.

History

Historically, Western medical ethics may be traced to guidelines on the duty of physicians in antiquity, such as the Hippocratic Oath, and early rabbinic and Christian teachings. In the medieval and early modern period, the field is indebted to Muslim medicine such as Ishaq bin Ali Rahawi (who wrote the Conduct of a Physician, the first book dedicated to medical ethics) and Muhammad ibn Zakariya ar-Razi (known as Rhazes in the West), Jewish thinkers such as Maimonides, Roman Catholic scholastic thinkers such as Thomas Aquinas, and the case-oriented analysis (casuistry) of Catholic moral theology. These intellectual traditions continue in Catholic, Islamic and Jewish medical ethics.

By the 18th and 19th centuries, medical ethics emerged as a more self-conscious discourse. For instance, authors such as Thomas Percival wrote about "medical jurisprudence" and reportedly coined the phrase "medical ethics." Percival's guidelines related to physician consultations have been criticized as being excessively protective of the home physician's reputation. Jeffrey Berlant is one such critic who considers Percival's codes of physician consultations as being an early example of the anti-competitive, "guild"-like nature of the physician community.[1, 2] In 1847, the American Medical Association adopted its first code of ethics, with this being based in large part upon Percival's work.[3] While the secularized field borrowed largely from Catholic medical ethics, in the 20th century a distinctively liberal Protestant approach was articulated by thinkers such as Joseph Fletcher. In the 1960s and 1970s, building upon liberal theory and procedural justice, much of the discourse of medical ethics went through a dramatic shift and largely reconfigured itself into bioethics.[4]

Since the 1970s, the growing influence of ethics in contemporary medicine can be seen in the increasing use of Institutional Review Boards to evaluate experiments on human subjects, the establishment of hospital ethics committees, the expansion of the role of clinician ethicists, and the integration of ethics into many medical school curricula.[5]

---

[1] Berlant, Jeffrey (1975). Profession and Monopoly: a study of medicine in the United States and Great Britain. University of California Press. ISBN 0520027345.
http://www.pubmedcentral.nih.gov/articlerender.fcgi?artid=108181
6.
[2] Percival, Thomas (1849). Medical ethics. John Henry Parker. pp. 49–57 esp section 8 pg.52.
http://books.google.com/?id=yVUEAAAAQAAJ&printsec=frontc
over&dq=medical+ethics.
[3] Lakhan SE, Hamlat E, McNamee T, Laird C (2009). "Time for a unified approach to medical ethics." Philosophy, Ethics, and Humanities in Medicine 4 (3): 13. doi:10.1186/1747-5341-4-13. PMC 2745426. PMID 19737406.
http://www.pubmedcentral.nih.gov/articlerender.fcgi?tool=pmcentr
ez&artid=2745426.
[4] Walter, Klein eds. The Story of Bioethics: From seminal works to contemporary explorations.
[5] Lakhan SE, Hamlat E, McNamee T, Laird C (2009). "Time for a unified approach to medical ethics." Philosophy, Ethics, and Humanities in Medicine 4 (3): 13. doi:10.1186/1747-5341-4-13. PMC

Values in Medical Ethics

Six of the values that commonly apply to medical ethics discussions are:

1. **Autonomy** - the patient has the right to refuse or choose their treatment. (*Voluntas aegroti suprema lex.*)

2. **Beneficence** - a practitioner should act in the best interest of the patient. (*Salus aegroti suprema lex.*)

3. **Non-maleficence** - "first, do no harm" (*primum non nocere*).

4. **Justice** - concerns the distribution of scarce health resources, and the decision of who gets what treatment (*fairness and equality*).

5. **Dignity** - the patient (and the person treating the patient) have the right to dignity.

6. **Truthfulness and honesty** - the concept of informed consent has increased in importance since the historical events of the Doctors' Trial of the Nuremberg trials and Tuskegee Syphilis Study.

Values such as these do not give answers as to how to handle a particular situation, but provide a useful framework for understanding conflicts.

When moral values are in conflict, the result may be an ethical dilemma or crisis. Sometimes, no good solution to a dilemma in medical ethics exists, and occasionally, the values of the medical community (i.e., the hospital and its staff) conflict with the

2745426. PMID 19737406.
http://www.pubmedcentral.nih.gov/articlerender.fcgi?tool=pmcentr ez&artid=2745426.

values of the individual patient, family, or larger non-medical community. Conflicts can also arise between health care providers, or among family members. Some argue for example, that the principles of autonomy and beneficence clash when patients refuse blood transfusions, considering them life-saving; and truth-telling was not emphasized to a large extent before the HIV era.

Army Medical Command

The U.S. Army Medical Command (MEDCOM) is a major command of the U.S. Army that provides command and control of the Army's fixed-facility medical, dental, and veterinary treatment facilities, providing preventive care, medical research and development and training institutions.

Structure and Subordinate Commands

MEDCOM is divided into Regional Medical Commands that oversee day-to-day operations in military treatment facilities, exercising command and control over the medical treatment facilities in their regions. There are currently five of these regional commands:

- Europe Regional Medical Command

- Southern Regional Medical Command

- Northern Regional Medical Command

- Pacific Regional Medical Command

- Western Regional Medical Command.

Additional subordinate commands of MEDCOM include:

- Army Medical Department Center & School (AMEDDC&S)

- U.S. Army Public Health Command (Provisional), (known as the U.S. Army Center for Health Promotion & Preventive Medicine prior to 1 October 2009 {USACHPPM or CHPPM})

- U.S. Army Medical Research and Materiel Command (USAMRMC)

- Warrior Transition Command (WTC)

- U.S. Army Dental Command (DENCOM)

Operations

In Garrison (Peacetime)

MEDCOM maintains day-to-day health care for soldiers, retired soldiers and the families of both. Despite the wide range of responsibilities involved in providing health care in traditional settings as well as on the battlefield, the Army Medical Department's quality of care compares very favorably with that of civilian health organizations, when measured by civilian standards. Many Army medical facilities report on their own quality-of-care standards on their individual Internet sites.

Deployments

When Army field hospitals deploy, most clinical professional and support personnel come from MEDCOM's fixed facilities. In addition to support of combat operations, deployments can be for humanitarian assistance, peacekeeping, and other stability and support operations. Under the Professional Officer Filler System (PROFIS), up to

26 percent of MEDCOM physicians and 43 percent of MEDCOM nurses are sent to field units during a full deployment. To replace PROFIS losses, Reserve units and Individual Mobilization Augmentees (non-unit reservists) are mobilized to work in medical treatment facilities. The department also provides trained medical specialists to the Army's combat medical units, which are assigned directly to combatant commanders.

Many Army Reserve and Army National Guard units deploy in support of the Army Medical Department. The Army depends heavily on its Reserve component for medical support—about 63 percent of the Army's medical forces are in the Reserve component.

Army Medical Department

The Army Medical Department of the U.S. Army (AMEDD) comprises the Army's six medical Special Branches (or "Corps") of officers and medical enlisted soldiers. It was established as the "Army Hospital" in July 1775 to coordinate the medical care required by the Continental Army during the Revolutionary War. The AMEDD is led by the Surgeon General of the U.S. Army, a lieutenant general.

The AMEDD is the U.S. Army's healthcare organization, not a U.S. Army command. The AMEDD is found in all three components of the Army: the Active Army, the U.S. Army Reserve, and the Army National Guard. Its headquarters are at Fort Sam Houston, San Antonio, Texas, which hosts the AMEDD Center and School. Equal numbers of AMEDD senior leaders can be found in Washington D.C., divided between the Pentagon and the Walter Reed Army Medical Center (WRAMC).

The Academy of Health Sciences, under the Army Medical Department Center & School, provides training to the officers and enlisted soldiers of the AMEDD. As a result of BRAC 2005, enlisted medical training was transferred to the new Medical Education and Training Campus, consolidating most military enlisted medical training at Fort Sam Houston.[6]

Medical Special Branches

- Medical Corps (MC)

- Nurse Corps (AN)

- Dental Corps (DC)

- Veterinary Corps (VC)

- Medical Service Corps (MS)

- Medical Specialist Corps (AMSC)

United States Army Training and Doctrine Command

Established 1 July 1973, the United States Army Training and Doctrine Command (TRADOC) is an army command of the United States Army headquartered at Fort Monroe, Virginia. It is charged with overseeing training of Army forces, the development of operational doctrine, and the development and procurement of new weapons systems. TRADOC operates 33 schools and centers at 16 Army installations. TRADOC schools conduct 2,734 courses (81 directly in support of mobilization)

---

[6] U.S. Army Medical Department AMEDD Center and School Portal available on the Internet at: http://www.cs.amedd.army.mil/. Additional information specific to the Fort Sam Houston consolidation is available n the Internet at: http://www.aetc.af.mil/shared/media/document/AFD-071026-035.pdf

and 373 language courses. The 2,734 courses include 503,164 seats for 434,424 soldiers; 34,675 other-service personnel; 7,824 international soldiers; and 26,241 civilians.[7]

TRADOC MissionThe official mission statement for TRADOC states:

> TRADOC develops the Army's Soldiers and Civilian leaders and designs, develops and integrates capabilities, concepts and doctrine in order to build a campaign-capable, expeditionary Army in support of joint warfighting capability through Army Force Generation (ARFORGEN).[8]

TRADOC is the official command component that is responsible for training and developing the United States Army.

TRADOC History

TRADOC was established as a major U.S. Army command on 1 July 1973. The new command, along with the U.S. Army Forces Command (FORSCOM), was created from the Continental Army Command (CONARC) located at Fort Monroe, VA. That action was the major innovation in the Army's post-Vietnam reorganization, in the face of realization that CONARC's obligations and span of control were too broad for efficient focus. The new organization functionally realigned the major Army commands in the continental United States. CONARC, and Headquarters, U.S. Army Combat Developments Command (CDC), situated at Fort Belvoir, VA, were discontinued, with TRADOC and FORSCOM at Fort Belvoir assuming the realigned missions. TRADOC assumed the combat

---

[7] TRADOC fact sheet available at:
http://www.tradoc.army.mil/about.htm
[8] TRADOC commander on ARFORGEN, and the US Army available at: http://www.tradoc.army.mil/about.htm

developments mission from CDC, took over the individual training mission formerly the responsibility of CONARC, and assumed command from CONARC of the major Army installations in the United States housing Army training center and Army branch schools. FORSCOM assumed CONARC's operational responsibility for the command and readiness of all divisions and corps in the continental U.S. and for the installations where they were based.

Joined under TRADOC, the major Army missions of individual training and combat developments each had its own lineage. The individual training responsibility had belonged, during World War II, to Headquarters Army Ground Forces (AGF). In 1946 numbered Army areas were established in the U.S. under AGF command. At that time, the AGF moved from Washington, D.C. to Fort Monroe, VA. In March 1948, the AGR was replaced at Fort Monroe with the new Office, Chief of Army Field Forces (OCAFF). OCAFF, however, did not command the training establishment. That function was exercised by Headquarters, Department of the Army through the numbered Armies to the corps, division, and Army Training Centers. In February 1955, HQ Continental Army Command (CONARC) replaced OCAFF, assuming its missions as well as the training missions from DA. In January, HQ CONARC was redesignated U.S. Continental Army Command. Combat developments emerged as a formal Army mission in the early 1950s, and OCAFF assumed that role in 1952. In 1955, CONARC assumed the mission. In 1962, HQ U.S. Army Combat Development Command (CDC) was established to bring the combat developments function under one major Army command.[9]

---

[9] TRADOC history available at:
http://www.tradoc.army.mil/about.htm

TRADOC Priorities

1. Leader Development
2. Initial Military Training
3. Concepts and Capabilities Integration
4. Human Capital Enterprise
5. Army Training and Learning Concept
6. Doctrine

Clinical Handbook

Supportive Care 1

This page intentionally left blank.

91W10
Advanced Individual
Training Course

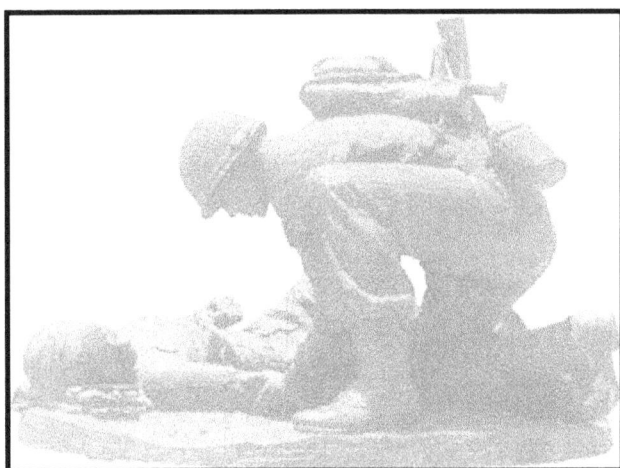

Clinical Handbook
Supportive Care

Department of the Army
Academy of Health Sciences
Fort Sam Houston, Texas 78234

TERMINAL LEARNING OBJECTIVE

Given a standard fully stocked M5 Bag or Combat Medic Vest System, IV administration equipment and fluids, oxygen, suction and ventilation equipment (if available) and glucometer. You encounter a casualty who has a metabolic and endocrine systems problem.

Principles of glucose metabolism

All body cells use glucose as an energy source
The brain requires a constant supply of glucose
The blood stream delivers glucose to the cells for use as energy
Insulin must be present for glucose to enter the cells
Glucose and insulin balance are necessary for effective metabolism and use of glucose as an energy source

Without insulin

(1)   Glucose cannot enter the cell from the bloodstream
(2)   Acids are formed when fat is used for energy needs and can lead to diabetic ketoacidosis

The three Ps of weight loss occur when glucose is not adequately metabolized. Frequently seen in undiagnosed diabetics.

(1)   Polyuria – The excess amount of glucose in the blood forces water into the bloodstream. The extra water is secreted as excess urine.
(2)   Polydipsia – increased thirst that results in increased water drinking. Secondary to increased volume of urine.
(3)   Polyphagia – The cells and tissues cannot utilize the sugar in the blood; therefore, the cells begin to starve. This starvation causes hunger and excessive eating.
(4)   Weight loss – The cells cannot use the sugar, so they break down fat and protein for energy causing weight loss

Assess the casualty for hypoglycemia and hyperglycemia

Hypoglycemia is a true medical emergency!

Hypoglycemia

(1)   Generally defined as a serum glucose level of less than 50 mg/dl
(2)   Signs and symptoms (tachycardia, cool, moist or clammy skin, dizziness, complaints of hunger) are consistent with the diagnosis
(3)   Signs and symptoms are resolved following glucose administration.

Causes of hypoglycemia

(1)   In an insulin-dependent diabetic is often the result of too much insulin, too little food, or both
(2)   A diabetic who has not eaten does not have enough dietary intake of glucose to use for a circulating level of insulin
(3)   Excessive exercise or exertion uses up the glucose energy stores
(4)   Vomiting or diarrhea depletes the body of fluids, electrolytes, and potential sources of glucose

Academy of Health Sciences
91W10
Treat Metabolic Endocrine Symptoms

Signs and symptoms of hypoglycemia
   (1)   Rapid onset - over a period of minutes
   (2)   Intense hunger
   (3)   Cold, pale, moist, or clammy skin
   (4)   Full, rapid pulse
   (5)   May appear intoxicated
   (6)   Dizziness and headache
   (7)   Copious saliva (drooling)
   (8)   Normal blood pressure
   (9)   Altered mental status and seizures are symptoms of severe hypoglycemia (blood glucose < 30 mg/dl)

Treatment and transport considerations for hypoglycemia
   (1)   Conscious patient
        (a)   Perform the initial assessment. Check for a medical alert identification
        (b)   Perform a focused history and physical exam and SAMPLE history
        (c)   Perform a D (dextrose) stick or Accucheck as per local protocol
        (d)   Administer oral glucose IAW local protocol if all three of the following are present:
            (i)   The patient has a history of diabetes
            (ii)   The patient's mental status is altered
            (iii)   The patient is awake enough to swallow
            (iv)   Dose - one glucose tube
        (e)   Adult - Place glucose on the tongue depressor between the cheek and the gum or self administer it between the cheek and the gum
        (f)   If oral glucose is not available, give granular sugar, honey, hard candy, or orange juice
        (g)   If a patient becomes unconscious, remove the tongue depressor and assure and open the airway
        (h)   Monitor and maintain airway
   (2)   Unconscious patient and/or inability to swallow

WARNING: DO NOT GIVE UNCONSCIOUS PATIENTS ANYTHING BY MOUTH!

        (a)   Initiate and maintain IV of normal saline (promotes excretion of keynote bodies)
        (b)   Administer pharmacological interventions
            (i)   50% Dextrose
            (ii)   Therapeutic effects: Rapidly restores blood sugar levels to normal in states of hypoglycemia
            (iii)   Indications: To treat suspected hypoglycemia or a coma of unknown cause
            (iv)   Contraindications: Intracranial hemorrhage, known stroke (CVA)

        (v)   Side effects: Will cause tissue necrosis if it infiltrates

        (vi)   How supplied: Prefilled syringes containing 50 cc of 50% dextrose (25 Grams)

        (vii)   Administration and dosage: Give through patent IV line. If possible obtain serum glucose prior to administration dosage is 50ml of 50% solution

    (c)   Treat patient like any other with an altered mental status

    (d)   Continue to monitor and maintain airway

    (e)   Administer oxygen, if available

    (f)   Start artificial ventilations if necessary

    (g)   Transport - Continue ongoing assessment en route.

(3)   Position patient - If the patient does not require artificial ventilations, place him in a lateral recumbent position in case s/he vomits

When cause is known, treat as though hypoglycemia; give sugar

    (1)   A patient in diabetic ketoacidosis will not be harmed by having sugar

    (2)   A patient in severe hypoglycemia will respond rapidly

    CAUTION: When a patient appears intoxicated, treat the patient as a diabetic emergency. Always check for underlying conditions. Never assume the patient is "only drunk."

Hyperglycemia

    (1)   Generally defined as a random blood glucose > 200 mg/dl or a fasting blood glucose > 140 mg/dl

Causes of hyperglycemia

    (1)   Undiagnosed/untreated diabetic condition

    (2)   Insulin not taken

    (3)   Overeating

    (4)   Infection that disrupts glucose/insulin balance

    (5)   Myocardial infarction (heart attack)

Signs and symptoms (Blood glucose 200-400 mg/dl)

    (1)   Patients are often asymptomatic. Increased blood glucose is found on incidental laboratory examination or a random self glucose test.

    (2)   Slow onset - occurs over a period of days or weeks

    (3)   Dry mouth

    (4)   Intense thirst

    (5)   Frequent urination

    (6)   Blurred vision

    (7)   Frequent infections

Signs and symptoms (Blood glucose > 400 mg/dl)

    (1)   Usually more dramatic presentation

    (2)   Intense thirst

    (3)   Abdominal pain

    (4)   Vomiting

    (5)   Progressive restlessness/confusion

    (6)   Respiration may be very deep and rapid (Kussmaul respirations)

(7)   Weak, rapid pulse
(8)   Warm, red, dry skin
(9)   Sunken eyes
(10)   Acetone breath (fruity odor)
(11)   May appear intoxicated
(12)   Normal to slightly low blood pressure

Treatment and transport considerations
(1)   Maintain an open airway
(2)   Administer a high concentration of O2, if available
(3)   Perform D (dextrose) stick or Accucheck per local protocol
(4)   Initiate and maintain an IV of Normal Saline
(5)   Transport immediately
(6)   Continuously monitor vital signs

WARNING: If untreated, hyperglycemia will eventually lead to diabetic
ketoacidosis. The metabolism of substances other than sugar
creates high levels of acid in the blood. THIS PROCESS CAN
LEAD TO DEATH.

Disorders of the Thyroid Gland
Common acute thyroid disorders include
(1)   Hyperthyroidism – presence of excess thyroid hormones in the blood
(2)   Thyrotoxicosis – a condition that reflects prolonged exposure of body
organs to excess thyroid hormones, with resultant changes in
structure and function. Thyrotoxicosis is generally caused by Grave's
Disease
(3)   Thyrotoxic Crisis – "Thyrotoxic Storm" life threatening emergency
characterized by hyperthermia, nervous symptoms, and rapid
metabolism
(4)   Hyperthyroidism – presence of inadequate thyroid hormones in the
blood
(5)   Myxedema – condition that reflects long-term inadequate levels of
thyroid hormones with resultant change in function and structure
(6)   Myxedema Coma – uncommon complication of myxedema that can
be fatal if respiratory depression occurs. Usually triggered by acute
infection, trauma, cold infection, exposure to CNS depressants such
as alcohol and drugs.

Thyrotoxicosis
(1)   Less serious than Thyroid Storm
(2)   Important causes of palpitations
(3)   Commonly caused by undiagnosed or untreated Graves' disease,
infectious process or surgery

Thyroid storm (more serious form of Thyrotoxicosis)
(1)   Medical emergency
- (a)   Elevated temperature (T>38.7⁰ C, but may be as high as 41 ⁰ C)
- (b)   CNS dysfunction (anxiety, emotional lability, delirium)
- (c)   Cardiovascular dysfunction
- (d)   Gastrointestinal dysfunction (nausea, vomiting, hyperdefecation or diarrhea, crampy abdominal pain)
- (e)   May mimic or complicate sepsis, sympathomimetic intoxication, or a drug withdrawal

Signs and symptoms
- (1)   Sinus tachycardia (heart rate > 100 bpm) is almost always present
- (2)   Heart rate may be fast and irregular
- (3)   Enlarged thyroid may be palpable
- (4)   Proptosis and other eye findings indicative of Graves' disease
- (5)   Brisk reflexes
- (6)   Anxiety
- (7)   Tremor
- (8)   Weakness
- (9)   Heat intolerance
- (10)   Weight loss
- (11)   Hyperdefecation
- (12)   Sweating
- (13)   Angina and congestive heart failure (CHF) may be present

Treatment considerations

NOTE: In most cases mild thyrotoxicosis is referred for outpatient evaluation and treatment.   If patient is symptomatic but not acutely ill, beta–adrenergic blockade with propranolol (slow 1 mg IV bolus may be administered in accordance with physicians' orders).

(1)   Emergency care for Thyroid storm
- (a)   Provide supportive care including cooling measures (ice packs, cooling blankets)
- (b)   Contact MD/PA immediately for specific guidance
- (c)   Initiate and maintain IV access and fluids
- (d)   Administer oxygen

(2)   Provide on-going management for Thyroid storm
- (a)   Monitor patient's response to treatment
- (b)   Monitor airway if unconscious
- (c)   Place patient in quiet, reassuring environment, if possible
- (d)   Maintain IV fluids as directed
- (e)   Evacuate for further treatment as required

(3)   It is imperative to consider other processes as precipitants of thyroid storm or as a primary cause of symptoms
- (a)   Infection
- (b)   Surgery
- (c)   Trauma
- (d)   Emotional stress

Hypothyroidism
Hypothyroidism-

A condition of decreased activity of the thyroid gland

    (1)   Body's normal rate of functioning slows causing mental and physical sluggishness

    (2)   Most severe form is called myxedema, which is a medical emergency

Risk factors

    (1)   Over 50 years old

    (2)   Female

    (3)   Obesity

    (4)   Thyroid surgery

    (h)   X-ray or radiation treatments to the neck

Signs and symptoms

    (1)   Physical Examination and X-Ray

          (a)   Enlarged thyroid on physical exam

          (b)   Delayed reflexes

          (c)   Slow heart rate

          (d)   Low blood pressure

          (e)   Low temperature

          (f)   Chest x-ray indicates an enlarged heart

    (2)   Early symptoms:

          (a)   Weakness

          (b)   Fatigue

          (c)   Cold Intolerance

          (d)   Constipation

          (e)   Weight gain

          (f)   Depression

          (g)   Joint or muscle

          (h)   Thin, brittle fingernails

          (i)   Coarse thick hair

          (j)   Pale color

    (3)   Late symptoms:

          (a)   Slow speech

          (b)   Dry flaky skin

          (c)   Thickening of the skin

          (d)   Puffy face, hands and feet

          (e)   Decreased taste and smell

          (f)   Thinning of eyebrows

          (g)   Hoarseness

          (h)   Menstrual disorders

Myxedema –
Untreated severe hypothyroidism

    (1)   Thickness of connective tissue in the skin and other tissues including the heart

    (2)   Most commonly seen in middle aged or elderly

(3)   Myxedema Coma is a medical emergency and is manifested by
        profound hypothermia, bradycardia, and respiratory depression
(4)   Treatment is supportive – maintain and monitor airway
(5)   Transport/evacuate to definitive care facility immediately
(6)   May be fatal if left untreated

TERMINAL LEARNING OBJECTIVE

Given a CMVS or M5 aid bag standard packing list, IV administration equipment and fluids, oxygen, suction and ventilation equipment (if available), selected medications, documentation forms. You encounter a suspected casualty complaining of neurological symptoms. No other injury (ies) is/are present.

Determine the cause and/or mechanism of injury
   Levels of Consciousness –
      Abnormal levels of consciousness may be associated with decreased or increased neurological activity, such as stupor, coma, delirium, or violent behavior. There may be partial to complete mental clouding or loss of consciousness.

   (1)   Frequent causes of altered levels of consciousness are cerebrovascular accident (CVA), drugs, poisons, metabolic illness, fever, head injury, subarachnoid hematoma (SAH), Subdural hematoma (SDH), and epidural hematoma

   (2)   The two major categories of altered levels of consciousness are stupor and coma
      (a)   Stupor ranges from partial to almost complete loss of consciousness
      (b)   Coma is complete unconsciousness from which the patient cannot be roused

   (3)   Emergency Management of Life-Threatening Neurological Problems
      (a)   Confirm an unconscious state
         (i)   Attempt to arouse the patient by pinching or shouting to rule out sleep or a simple faint
      (b)   Secure the airway
      (c)   Give supplemental oxygen, if needed
      (d)   Establish adequacy of ventilation
         (i)   If respirations are slow or diminished, begin assisted ventilation
      (e)   Establish circulation - Begin CPR, if needed. Obtain vital signs, and treat shock, if present.
      (f)   Obtain description of the onset of illness or injury and a history of chronic illnesses e.g. diabetes, hypertension, drug abuse, chronic headaches
      (g)   Perform a rapid physical examination, utilizing the Glasgow Coma Scale

   (4)   The Glasgow Coma Scale
      (a)   Widely used method of evaluating the level of consciousness
      (b)   Glasgow Coma Scale assigns a numerical score to the patient's responses in three categories
         (i)   Eye opening
         (ii)   Best motor response
         (iii)   Best verbal response
      (c)   Repeat assessment frequently to assess for changes
      (d)   Assess the patient's score in each category, and total the scores of the tree categories.

(5)   Treatment - the immediate objective of emergency treatment and stabilization is to maintain life until a specific diagnosis can be made. **DONT** Protocol:

    (a)   **D**extrose
    (b)   **O**xygen
    (c)   **N**arcan
    (d)   Thiamin

Assess a casualty in a field setting using the Glasgow Coma Scale
Seek an appropriate location to conduct the neurological status exam
(1)   In a hostile zone
    (a)   Move the casualty to an area that provides adequate cover and concealment
    (b)   As with all injuries a primary survey must be conducted focusing on the ABC's and stabilizing life-threatening injuries before any type of assessment is started
    (c)   Time and Circumstances may not permit a full neurological assessment and in fact may dictate that the soldier medic move on to the next casualty after treating for life threatening injuries
    (d)   Assess the casualty using the Glasgow Coma Scale

Assess a patient with neurological symptoms in a clinical setting
A clinical environment lends itself to the conduct of a full neurological assessment.
Seek an appropriate setting to conduct the neurological status exam.
(1)   Use a well-lit room
(2)   Free of distractions
(3)   If available, question family and friends

Assess mental status and speech
(1)   Determine level of consciousness
    (a)   Normal
    (b)   Drowsiness
    (c)   Stupor
    (d)   Coma
(2)   Observe posture and motor behavior
    (a)   Gait
    (b)   Gestures
    (c)   Mannerisms
    (d)   Speed of movement - fast, normal, and slow
    (e)   Over or under active
    (f)   Purposeful or disorganized
(3)   Observe dress, grooming, and personal hygiene
    (a)   Appropriately dressed for age, social status
    (b)   Cleanliness
    (c)   Hair, teeth, and nail care
(4)   Observe facial expressions
    (a)   Appropriate to topics being discussed
    (b)   Describe
        (i)   Alert
        (ii)   Tense

        (iii)   Worried
        (iv)   Sad
        (v)   Happy
        (vi)   Angry
        (vii)   Laughing

(5)   Observe and record the patient's manner, affect, and relationship to persons and things
      (a)   Describe (afraid, seeking help, evasive, etc.)
      (b)   Affect- is the patient's voice, facial expression, and movement appropriate to topic being discussed?

Observe speech and language for
(1)   Quantity
(2)   Rate
(3)   Volume - rapid and loud, mania, soft and low

Observe Mood - as reported by patient
(1)   Intensity
(2)   Duration
(3)   Appropriate to circumstances

Observe thought and perceptions – are the patient's perceptions appropriate to the situation?

Memory and orientation
(1)   Orientation
      (a)   person - does pt know who he/she is
      (b)   place - location, where he/she lives
      (c)   time - day of week, date, time of day
(2)   Attention- does the patient answer appropriately?
(3)   Remote memory - place of birth, where he/she is from
(4)   Recent memory - questions related to the presenting problem. (the days weather, appointment time, etc.)

Suicidal and homicidal patients
(1)   MUST be evaluated by a Medical Officer (MO)
(2)   Most are not mentally ill, but overwhelmed by life stressors

Summary/Assessment of Mental Status
(1)   Summary of findings/conclusions
(2)   The mental exam is the psychiatric counterpart of the physical exam

General approach to the neurologic exam
(1)   Organize exam into 5 basic areas
      (a)   mental status/speech -as previously discussed
      (b)   cranial nerves
      (c)   cerebellar
      (d)   motor
      (e)   sensory
      (f)   reflexes

Techniques of examination
- (1) Mental status and speech- as described above
- (2) Cranial nerves
  - (a) Mnemonics for remembering nerves (1st letter stands for first letter of nerve)
    - (i) On Old Olympus Towering Tops, A Finn And German Viewed Some Hops (Tests the olfactory, optic, oculomotor, trochlear, trigeminal, abducens, facial, acoustic, glossopharyngeal, vagus, spinal accessory, & hypoglossal)
  - (b) Cranial Nerve I (CN-I): Olfactory
    - (i) Sense of smell
    - (ii) Test by holding familiar items under the patient's nose with their eyes closed. Clamp each nostril testing each one separately.
  - (c) Cranial nerve II (CN-II): Optic
    - (i) Vision sense
    - (ii) Tests visual acuity, visual fields, peripheral vision, and fundoscopic exam
  - (d) Cranial nerves III, IV, & VI: Oculomotor = CN-III, Trochlear = CN-IV, Abducens = CN-VI
    - (i) Function
      - * CN-III - extraocular muscle movement, pupillary light accommodation and consensual reflexes, and elevation of eyelid
      - * CN-IV – extraocular muscle movement
      - * CN-VI – extraocular muscle movement
    - (ii) Test for extraocular muscle movement by:
      - * Holding a small object in front of patient
      - * Have patient follow object as it is moved through the 6 cardinal positions of gaze
    - (iii) Test for size and shape of pupils and pupillary reaction to light
  - (e) Fifth cranial nerve (CN-V): Trigeminal nerve
    - (i) Function
      - * Motor - temporal, and masseter muscles along with lateral movement of the jaw
      - * Sensory - three separate distributions, V-1 = to the forehead, V-2= to the cheeks, V-3 = to the chin
    - (ii) Test function
      - * Test motor function by having patient clench teeth and move jaw side to

side. Palpate strength of muscle
contraction. Feel contraction of
temporal muscles.

* Test sharp/dull sensation with a safety
pin and light touch to forehead,
cheeks, and chin on both sides

(f) 7th cranial nerve (CN-VII): Facial nerve
(i) Function
* Motor - muscle of facial expression
(ii) Test function
* Inspect face for symmetry or abnormal
movements
* Have patient raise eyebrows, frown,
close eyes tightly (and test strength by
trying to open them with your fingers).
Show upper and lower teeth, smile
and puff out cheeks

(g) 8th cranial nerve (CN-VIII): Vestibulocochlear
(i) Function
* Hearing
(ii) Test hearing
* Snap fingers in front of each ear to
assess gross hearing function

(h) 9th & 10th cranial nerves: CN-IX Glossopharyngeal, CN-X
Vagus
(i) Function
* CN-IX: sensory - posterior ear
drum/canal, pharynx. Motor -
pharynx.
* CN-X: sensory - pharynx & larynx.
Motor - soft palate, pharynx, and
larynx/vocal cords.
(ii) Test for
* Vocal quality
* Observe upward movement of
posterior oropharynx and symmetry
* Stimulate gag reflex on each side with
cotton swab
* Ability to elevate palate

(i) 11th cranial nerve (CN-XI): Spinal accessory nerve
(i) Function
* Motor - upper portion of
sternocleidomastoid and trapezius
muscles
(ii) Test for
* Ability to turn head side to side
* Ability to shrug shoulders upwards
against resistance

(j) 12th cranial nerve (CN-XII): Hypoglossal nerve
(i) Function

                        *   Motor to tongue

(ii)   Test for function
* Symmetry, atrophy, or fasciculations
* Have patient move tongue side to side
* Have patient stick tongue out, should not deviate from midline

(3)   Cerebellar
    (a)   Inspection
        (i)   Ask pt to walk across room, down hall, turn and come back
        (ii)   Observe posture
        (iii)   Note presence of involuntary movements or swaying
        (iv)   Special maneuvers
* Heel to toe walking in a straight line
* Walk on toes
* Walk on heels
* Romberg test - have pt stand with heels and feet together, arms at sides and eyes closed. Observe for loss of position sense and tendency to fall.
* Hop in place on each foot. This indicates intact lower extremity motor systems, cerebellar function and position sense.

(4)   Motor
        (a)   Assessment of muscle tone
        (i)   Passive range of motion (with pt relaxed, perform range of motion to limbs for each joint.)
    (b)   Testing muscle strength
        (i)   Test specific motor groups
        (ii)   Have patient actively resist your attempts to flex or extend across specific joints
        (iii)   Grade muscle strength on scale of 0-5
* 0 = no muscular contraction noted
* 1 = barely detectable flicker of contraction
* 2 = active movement of body part with gravity
* 3 = active movement against gravity
* 4 = active movement against gravity with some resistance
* 5 = active movement against full resistance & without any evidence of fatigue (normal muscle strength)

(5)   Sensory
    (a)   General principles
        (i)   Note ability to perceive stimulus
        (ii)   Compare sensation

        (iii)   Scatter stimuli to cover most major peripheral
                      nerves
        (iv)   Vary the placement of your exam
        (v)   Map areas of altered sensation by proceeding in
                      a stepwise fashion outwards until patient detects
                      change

(b)   Pain
        (i)   Use sharp/dull areas of a safety pin
        (ii)   Use light pressure

(c)   Light touch
        (i)   Touch skin lightly with wisp of cotton and ask
                      patient to respond
        (ii)   Compare sides

(6)   Reflexes
     (a)   Graded on a 0-4 scale
        (i)   Four plus (4+) = very brisk, hyperactive
        (ii)   Three plus (3+) = brisker than normal
        (iii)   Two plus (2+) = normal
        (iv)   One plus (1+) = diminished
        (v)   Zero (0) = absent, no response

Assessment of Patient with Specific Neurological Symptoms

Dizziness and Vertigo

(1)   Dizziness is a perception of self-motion or a distortion of gravitational orientation. Dizziness is not a defined disease, but a sensory syndrome that may be produced by numerous diseases.

(2)   Vertigo is an illusionary sensation of motion or having objects move around the patient

(3)   Dizziness and vertigo should be distinguished from imbalance and syncope (loss of consciousness)

(4)   Symptoms - the patient is usually in an upright position when an acute attack occurs. They may experience:
     (a)   Motor weakness
     (b)   Epigastric distress
     (c)   Perspiration
     (d)   Restlessness
     (d)   Nausea and vomiting
     (e)   Tinnitus (ringing in the ears)
     (h)   Patients commonly have recurrent episodes

(5)   Treatment
     (a)   Management of the patient depends on the disease causing the dizziness or vertigo. All patients MUST have a full cardiac and neurological examination during initial assessment. Dizziness and vertigo are common symptoms in the elderly with cardiac disease.
     (b)   Initial stabilization utilizing a Glasgow Coma Scale should be performed if the patient is rapidly deteriorating. Serial neurological examinations should be performed while transporting patient to a MD/PA to assess.

(c)   All patients with an acute onset of dizziness or vertigo need to be evaluated by an MD/PA

Headaches –
Headaches are the most common pain complaint in patients. The number of different types of headache, their causes, signs, symptoms and treatments often make headache difficult to diagnose and treat. They may be caused by, tension, tumors, trauma, or any number of other causes. The following are the more common types of headaches:

(1)   Tension - These headaches are caused by spasm or contraction of muscles or adjacent structures, or they may be associated with fatigue or emotional stress. The muscles attached to the occiput and temple are the most frequently involved. These muscles will be tender to palpation

      (a)   Symptoms
            (i)   Feeling of pressure or a bandlike constriction around head. Pain is almost always bilateral
            (ii)   Not associated with vomiting. Nausea may be present
            (iii)   Patient with a tension headache will have a normal neurological examination

      (b)   Treatment - general measures consist of:
            (i)   Analgesics
            (ii)   Rest
            (iii)   Relaxation
            (iv)   Massage, and heat applied to the involved musculature
            (v)   Oral fluid hydration usually benefits headache patients- particularly in a field environment

(2)   Migraine - this type of headache is characterized by a paroxysmal attack often preceded by psychological or visual disturbance that is followed by drowsiness. Migraine headaches are believed to be the result of inflammatory vascular changes.

      (a)   Symptoms
            (i)   Specific symptoms vary with the type of migraine
            (ii)   Before the onset of a migraine headache, some patients experience a prodrome or aura. Visual auras are the most common (flashing lights or diminished vision)
            (iii)   Pain is usually unilateral- sometimes severe
            (iv)   Nausea, vomiting, photophobia (intolerance to light), phonophobia (intolerance to loud noise) may occur
            (v)   Patients may have an ill appearance
            (vi)   Other than an ill appearance, the physical examination are normal

      (b)   Often there is a family history of migraines, and the frequency of attacks may vary from daily to once every few years

(c)   Treatment Overview
(i)   Treatment of migraine is a three-faceted
        approach: abortive (at the immediate onset of
        headache); interval (during the headache) and
        prophylactic (to prevent future headaches
(ii)   Abortive therapy is useful during the aura or at
        the start of a migraine. Various oral, nasal and
        subcutaneous medications (i.e. Cafergot,
        Imitrex) can be used as abortive therapy.
(iii)   Interval therapy is directed at treating the
        migraine headache. Medications include
        analgesics (Toradol), antiemetics (Phenergan,
        Compazine) and abortive agents as above
(iv)   Prophylactic therapy is aimed at prevention or
        reduction of the frequency and severity of
        headaches. Numerous categories of
        medications are used for this.
(d)   Treatment of an Acute Migraine
(i)   Place the patient on bed rest in a darkened
        room, withhold any food or drink and initiate IV
        hydration. Fluids are helpful in migraine
        headaches
(ii)   Utilize the medications described above for
        abortive or interval therapy as ordered by a
        MD/PA
(iii)   Serial neurological evaluations should be
        performed. Reassess the patient after each
        medication is given
(iv)   Evacuate the patient to be evaluated by an
        MD/PA for assessment and management

Seizures –
A seizure is defined as the behavioral manifestation of abnormal neurologic
activity. Seizures are usually accompanied by altered levels of consciousness.
Epilepsy is a pattern of two or more recurrent seizures. In 75% of nontraumatic
seizures the cause is unknown. There are two types of seizure classifications
(1)   The two major classifications are:
        (a)   Generalized- bilateral foci that begin simultaneously
        (b)   Partial- single focus in cerebrum
(2)   Generalized Seizures
        (a)   Most commonly encountered and include the petit mal and
                grand mal types
        (b)   Typical generalized seizure
                (i)   Signs and symptoms
                        *   The patient may fall down and cry out,
                                lose bladder and bowel control, and
                                froth at the mouth
                        *   There is convulsive movement of the
                                body, dyspnea, and cyanosis

           *   Often the patient bites the tongue and, if not completely unconscious, will be confused and disoriented. The seizure usually lasts 2 to 5 minutes.

           *   A period of deep sleep is common after the seizure, and the patient will complain of muscle soreness and stiffness upon awakening

(ii)   Treatment - immediate treatment is aimed at airway, breathing, and circulation (ABC's) while preventing the patient from injuring him or herself. The second goal is identification of the seizure cause

           *   Do not use rigid restraints (may cause fractures) or insert objects into the patient's mouth during a seizure

           *   Never leave the patient alone. Protect the patient from further injury until seizure ends

           *   Loosen the clothing around the neck, and turn the head to the side to prevent aspiration of saliva and mucus

           *   Administer an anticonvulsant, such as Ativan 1-2 mg, or diazepam (Valium) 5-10 mg IV over 1-2 minutes. Give Valium only in the presence of active seizures. The objective of drug therapy is complete suppression of symptoms

           *   Refer the patient immediately to an MD/PA for evaluation. Perform serial neurological examinations during transport

Cerebrovascular Accident (Stroke)
    (1)   Strokes are caused by destruction of brain matter by intracerebral hemorrhage, thrombosis, embolism, or vascular insufficiency
    (2)   Stroke presentation is varied, depending on the area of brain that is involved. Symptoms include:
        (a)   Headache
        (b)   Nausea
        (c)   Vomiting
        (d)   Convulsions
        (e)   Coma
        (f)   Consciousness may not always be altered
        (g)   The patient may experience speech disturbances
        (h)   Confusion
        (i)   Loss of memory

	(j)	Reduction of sensation, and paralysis of extremities or of a complete side of the body
	(k)	The onset may be sudden and violent, with the patient falling into an immediate coma and exhibiting stertorous breathing
	(l)	Death from a serious stroke may result in a few minutes to a few days
(3)	Treatment	
	(a)	ABC's
	(b)	Administer IV fluids (TKO)
	(c)	Place the patient on immediate and strict bed rest
	(d)	Keep head elevated 30 degrees
	(e)	Evacuate the patient for hospitalization immediately
	(f)	Cardiac monitoring, if available
	(g)	Serial neurological examinations during transport

Subarachnoid Hemorrhage (SAH) –
Characterized by sudden bleeding into the subarachnoid space that may be the result of trauma or a ruptured aneurysm

(1)	Symptoms - before the aneurysm ruptures	
	(a)	The aneurysm applies pressure to nerves that will manifest as headaches, ocular palsies, diplopia, facial pain, and a diminished visual field
	(b)	After rupture, severe headache
	(c)	Nausea
	(d)	Vomiting
	(e)	Stiffness of the neck
	(f)	Positive Kernig's sign
		(i) A diagnostic meningeal sign marked by loss of the ability of a supine patient to completely straighten the leg when it is fully flexed at the knee and hip
		(ii) Pain in the lower back and resistance to straightening the leg constitutes a positive Kernig's sign
	(g)	Bilateral Babinski's reflex is usually present
		(i) Dorsiflexion of the big toe with extension and fanning of the other toes elicited by firmly stroking the lateral aspect of the sole of the foot
	(h)	The consciousness of the patient may or may not be affected, and the blood pressure is often elevated
(2)	Treatment	
	(a)	ABC's
	(b)	Keep the patient at rest
	(c)	IV hydration (TKO)
	(d)	Avoid any medications
	(e)	Evacuate the patient immediately
	(f)	Cardiac monitoring
	(g)	Serial neurological examinations during transport

Subdural hematoma-

Caused by the rupture of a cerebral vein. They may be caused by trauma, tumors or a medication side effect (i.e. anticoagulants). There may be a loss of consciousness at the time of the injury followed by an asymptomatic period that may last for several hours to days

(1)   Signs and symptoms the patient may have later

        (a)   Increased intracranial pressure as described above

        (b)   About one half of all persons with subdural hematoma will experience facial muscle weakness

(2)   Treatment

        (a)   Ensure that the patient has a patent airway

        (b)   Oxygen, if available

        (c)   Cardiac monitoring, if available

        (d)   Serial neurological examinations during transport

        (f)   Evacuate the patient immediately

Epidural Hematoma –

Result of blood collecting in the potential space between the skull and the dura mater. Most (80 to 90 percent) result from blunt trauma to the temporal of temporoparietal area with an associated skull fracture and middle meningeal arterial disruption.

(1)   The classic history of an epidural hematoma is for the patient to experience immediate loss of consciousness after significant blunt head trauma. The patient then awakens and has a lucent period prior to again falling unconscious as the hematoma expands.

(2)   This "classic" syndrome occurs in only about 20 percent of cases. The majority of patients either never looses consciousness or never regains consciousness after the injury.

(3)   Signs and Symptoms

        (a)   Increase intracranial pressure as previously described

        (b)   Neurological status/mental status may change rapidly due to the high pressure arterial bleeding of an epidural hematoma and can lead to herniation. The sequence of bleeding and herniation usually occurs within hours.

(4)   Treatment

        (a)   Ensure open, patent airway

        (b)   Assist with ventilations, as needed

        (c)   Administer oxygen, if available

        (d)   Cardiac monitoring, if available

        (e)   Elevate head of body 30 degrees

        (f)   Serial neurological examinations during transport

        (g)   Evacuate the patient immediately

Herniated Disk –

In most cases, herniation or rupture of an intervertebral disk is the result of trauma. It may occur with sudden straining of the back in an odd position or while lifting in the trunk flex position. Herniation may occur immediately (acute trauma) or may take years to occur (repetitive trauma). Most herniation occurs in the lumbosacral area but may also occur in the cervical or thoracic regions.

(1)   Signs and symptoms

          (a)   Over 90 percent of all herniated disks occur at the fourth or fifth lumbar interspace
          (b)   There is pain upon palpation of the affected area
          (c)   The patient will have a limited range of motion
          (d)   The posture of the spine will be abnormal due to the loss of curvature of the spine
          (e)   The patient may exhibit mild weakness of the foot or extensor areas of the great toe
          (f)   There may be impaired sensations of pain or touch, and coughing or sneezing may cause radiation of the pain to the calf

(2)   Treatment
          (a)   Place the patient on bed rest with a backboard and administer analgesics for pain
          (b)   Prevent the patient from using any physical effort
          (c)   Applications of heat to the area of tenderness is beneficial
          (d)   Definitive treatment of herniated disks will occasionally require surgery. Most herniated discs can be managed medically, with rest and medications.
          (e)   Evacuate the patient as soon as possible

Refer to further medical care
Treatment for neurological symptoms
    May take many forms, which are beyond the scope of the soldier medic
Several emergency medical procedures-,
    Soldier medic can perform to minimize and or prevent further injury in trauma cases, and instances where the cause of injury is not obvious

(1)   Ensure that the casualty is removed from the source of injury and is stabilized, focusing on the ABC's and that life threatening injuries are treated promptly
(3)   Treat an unconscious casualty as having a potential neck or spinal injury. Immobilize and do not move the casualty unless absolutely necessary
(2)   If fractures of the spine are suspected in-line stabilization of the spine is maintained and the casualty is immobilized as necessary
(4)   If fractures of the skull are suspected that the casualty is placed in a position where the head is elevated at least 30 degrees unless other injuries prohibit that position
(5)   Avoid the use of pain medications that are CNS depressants
(6)   Evacuate the casualty a timely manner to the next level of care
(7)   Provide on going care to maintain the casualty's condition or prevent the condition from getting worse
(8)   As the situation permits document as much information as is available to send along with the casualty, so that more definitive medical care can be administered

TERMINAL LEARNING OBJECTIVE

Given a standard fully stocked Combat Medic Vest System (CMVS) or fully stocked M5 Bag, IV administration equipment and fluids, oxygen, suction and ventilation equipment (if available), selected medications, and documentation forms. You encounter a casualty complaining of cardio-pulmonary symptoms. No other injury(ies) is/are present. NBC agents have been ruled out

Assess Cardiac Compromise
Primary assessment
- (1) Ensure open airway
- (2) Assess breathing
- (3) Assess circulation
  - (a) If pulse is present, continue assessment
  - (b) If no pulse, begin CPR

Secondary assessment (specific to cardiopulmonary symptoms)
- (1) Recognize signs of cardiac compromise
  - (a) Squeezing, dull pressure, chest pain commonly radiating down arms or to the jaw
  - (b) Sudden onset of sweating
  - (c) Difficulty breathing (dyspnea)
  - (d) Anxiety, irritability
  - (e) Feeling of impending doom
  - (f) Nausea/vomiting
  - (g) Unresponsive to stimuli
- (2) Assess vital signs
  - (a) Respirations
  - (b) Pulse
  - (c) Blood pressure
  - (d) Temperature
  - (e) Pulse oximetry
- (3) Focused history
  - (a) Onset of symptoms
    - (i) Sudden
    - (ii) Gradual over time
    - (iii) Known cause or "trigger"
  - (b) Duration of symptoms
    - (i) Constant
    - (ii) Recurrent
  - (c) Pain on inspiration
  - (d) Length of time
  - (e) Fever
  - (f) Smoking history
  - (g) Past medical history of associated diseases
- (4) Assess location and level of pain
  - (a) Use acronym: OPQRST
    - (i) Onset
    - (ii) Provocation
    - (iii) Quality

(iv)   Radiation
(v)   Severity
(vi)   Time
(b)   Apply pain scale
     (i)   0 = no pain
     (ii)   10 = worst pain

Assess specific cardiovascular disease/disorder

(1)   Angina pectoris
     (a)   Sudden chest pain caused by lack of oxygen supply to a portion of heart muscle
     (b)   Reduced blood flow to heart muscle usually due to coronary artery disease
     (c)   Concurrent with or following:
          (i)   Physical activity
          (ii)   Stress
          (iii)   Heavy meals
          (iv)   Exposure to cold
          (v)   Windy weather
     (d)   Signs and symptoms
          (i)   Pain, pressure, tightness, or squeezing feeling in chest area lasting 3-5 minutes
          (ii)   Radiation of pain to neck, jaw, teeth, shoulder, arms, upper back, or abdomen
          (iii)   Shortness of breath
          (iv)   Weakness
          (v)   Nausea/indigestion
          (vi)   Sweating
(2)   Acute myocardial infarction (AMI)
     (a)   Death of a portion of the myocardium caused by inadequate blood/oxygen supply through the coronary arteries
     (b)   Causes include:
          (i)   Inadequate blood supply through the coronary arteries long enough in duration that myocardium is damaged from oxygen starvation
          (ii)   Damage of myocardium causes disruption of normal electrical conduction, resulting in irregular and/or ineffective heart activity
          (iii)   Blood supply may be reduced or stopped by: coronary artery spasm, embolus, arteriosclerosis, and atherosclerosis
     (c)   Signs and symptoms
     (i)   Some or all signs and symptoms of angina pectoris
          (ii)   Pain may be intermittent (come and go)
          (iii)   Duration of pain may be 30 minutes to several hours
          (iv)   Pain may occur while at rest
          (v)   Rest and/or nitroglycerin do not relieve pain

                    (vi)   Signs of shock
                    (vii)   Dyspnea
                    (viii)   Anxiety, irritability, or denial

(3)   Congestive Heart Failure (CHF)

      (a)   Failure of heart to pump blood adequately to maintain tissue perfusion

      (b)   Causes include:
                    (i)   Diseased heart valves
                    (ii)   Hypertension
                    (iii)   Obstructive pulmonary disease
                    (iv)   Ineffective pumping of left ventricle. Causes blood to back up into pulmonary circulation, resulting in congestion in the lungs. Can progress to pulmonary edema (an accumulation of fluid in lung tissues and alveoli)
                    (v)   Ineffective pumping of the right ventricle. Causes blood to back up into the systemic circulation, causing edema in hands, lower extremities, and sacral area, and distention of jugular veins.

      (c)   Signs and symptoms
                    (i)   Agitation
                    (ii)   Tachycardia
                    (iii)   Dyspnea with shallow and labored respirations
                    (iv)   Orthopnea - an abnormal condition in which a person must sit or stand to breathe deeply or comfortably
                    (v)   Noisy respirations
                    (vi)   Edema in extremities
                    (vii)   Diaphoresis
                    (viii)   Possible chest pain
                    (ix)   Distended neck veins
                    (x)   Upright posture

Provide Care for Cardiac Compromise

Primary assessment

(1)   Assess airway - ensure open airway
(2)   Assess breathing - ensure adequate ventilation
(v)   Assess circulation

Manage patient with known cardiac history

(1)   Place patient in position of comfort and in a quiet environment
(2)   Apply oxygen, as indicated
(3)   Apply cardiac monitor, if available
(4)   Minimize patient exertion
      (a)   Use appropriate transfer procedures
      (b)   Do NOT allow patient to walk to stretcher or down steps
(5)   Loosen restrictive clothing
(6)   IV access before administering nitroglycerin

(7)   Administer NTG as directed by MD/PA (See LP C191W063, Medication administration)

    (a)   Reassess patient history

    (b)   If nitro is not prescribed to that patient, gain permission from MD/PA or follow local SOP

    (c)   Ensure systolic blood pressure is 100 or above

    (d)   Administration

        (i)   Dose is one tablet or spray under tongue

        (ii)   Have patient keep mouth closed until dissolved and absorbed

        (iii)   Verify effectiveness - Patient should report burning sensation under tongue

(8)   Initiate cardiac monitoring (See LP C191W059, Cardiac monitoring)

    (a)   Placement of electrodes (12-lead EKG)

        (i)   Arms - anterior forearm or biceps

        (ii)   Legs - medial aspect of lower leg

        (iii)   Chest position

            *   V1 - fourth intercostal space, right sternal

            *   V2 - fourth intercostal space, left sternal

            *   V3 - midway between V2 and V4

            *   V4 - fifth intercostal space, midclavicular line

            *   V5 - same level as V4, anterior axillary line

            *   V6 - same level as V4 and V5 - midaxillary line

        (iv)   Ensure patient information has been entered

        (v)   Check leads for contact

        (vi)   Record as needed

Use AED, if needed

    (1)   Reassess patient's unresponsiveness

    (2)   Begin or continue CPR efforts

    (3)   Deliver shock

        (a)   Turn on power

        (b)   Attach device

            (i)   One pad to right of sternum just below the clavicle

            (ii)   Other to left of precordium

        (c)   Initiate analysis of rhythm

        (d)   Deliver shock in a series of three as indicated by AED

        (e)   Check for pulse after three shocks

    (4)   Reassess vital signs

Perform ongoing management

    (1)   Monitor vitals signs every 3-5 minutes

    (2)   Initiate CPR as needed

    (3)   Prepare to provide artificial respiration as needed

    (4)   Run EKG as indicated by MD/PA

Assess Respiratory Symptoms
Primary assessment
    (1)   Assess airway - ensure open airway
    (2)   Assess breathing - ensure adequate ventilation
    (3)   Assess circulation
            (a)   If pulse is present, continue assessment
            If no pulse, begin CPR

Secondary assessment (specific to pulmonary symptoms)
    (1)   Assuming ABCs are intact, begin AMPLE history
            (a)   Allergies
            (b)   Medications
            (c)   Past medical history
                    (i)   Asthma
                    (ii)   Heart disease
                    (iii)   Emphysema
                    (iv)   Smoking history
            (d)   Last oral intake
            (e)   Events leading to onset, consider asking:
                    (i)   Onset of symptoms
                        *   Sudden?
                        *   Gradual over time?
                        *   Known cause or "trigger"?
                    (ii)   Duration of symptoms
                        *   Constant?
                        *   Recurrent?
                    (iii)   Fever? Chills?
                    (iv)   Chest pain? Shortness of breath? Difficulty breathing?
                    (iii)   Have you had a cough?
                    *   Productive or non-productive?
                    *   Color of sputum?
                    (iv)   Other symptoms, such as nausea and vomiting?
    (2)   Assess vital signs
            (a)   Respirations
            (b)   Pulse
            (c)   Blood pressure
            (d)   Temperature
            (e)   Pulse oximetry
    (3)   Assess patient complaints
            (a)   When did the medical problems start?
            (b)   What are the medical problems?
            (c)   Duration of symptoms
                    (i)   Constant
                    (ii)   Recurrent
    (4)   Inspect chest
            (a)   Use of accessory muscles and sternal or muscle retraction
            (b)   Skin color

        (c)   Flaring of nares
        (d)   Difficulty breathing or periods of apnea
        (e)   Splinting the chest
        (f)   Stridor
        (g)   Productive cough
        (h)   Altered mechanical effort
                (i)   Limited rise and fall of chest
                (ii)   Gasping
                (iii)   Pursed lips
                (iv)   Chest wall paradoxical motion
        (i)   Medical - physiological barriers
                (i)   Pneumonia
                (ii)   Pulmonary edema
                (iii)   Chronic Obstructive Pulmonary Disease (COPD)
(5)   Palpate the chest
        (a)   Tenderness
        (b)   Pain
        (c)   Crepitus
        (d)   Skin temperature
(6)   Auscultate the lungs
        (a)   Evaluate both inspiration and expiration
        (b)   Wheezing
        (c)   Rhonchi, rales
        (d)   Absence of breath sounds

Provide Care for Respiratory Illness
Assessment findings
        (1)   Signs of severe respiratory impairment
        (2)   Rapid, shallow and short breaths
        (3)   Decrease lung sounds and/or wheezing
Care for respiratory symptoms
        (1)   Place patient in position of comfort and in a quiet environment
        (2)   Apply oxygen, as indicated
        (3)   Minimize patient exertion
                (a)   Use appropriate transfer procedures
                (b)   Do NOT allow patient to walk to stretcher or down steps
        (4)   Loosen restrictive clothing
        (5)   IV access, if indicated
        (6)   Cardiac monitoring, if patient has shortness of breath or chest pain

Upper respiratory infection
        (1)   Contagious viral infections of the upper respiratory tract
        (2)   Common symptoms include:
                (a)   Inflammation of the mucous membranes
                       (i)   Nasal congestion
                       (ii)   Runny nose
                (b)   Sneezing
                (c)   Sore throat
                (d)   Coughing

    (3)   Provide care - supportive measures
         (a)   Consider pain relievers
         (b)   Drink plenty of fluid
         (c)   Rest

Pharyngitis
    (1)   Most often caused by viral infections. May be cause by bacteria, such as group A streptococcus, which is commonly termed strep throat.
    (2)   Symptoms include:
         (a)   Sore throat
         (b)   Difficulty swallowing
         (c)   Fever
         (d)   Swollen lymph nodes
         (e)   Exudate on tonsils
         (f)   Beefy red throat
    (3)   Provide care
         (a)   For viral infections, treatment is to relieve symptoms only
              (i)   Consider pain relievers for pain
              (ii)   Consider gargle with warm salt water
         (b)   Bacterial pharyngitis is treated with antibiotics

Bronchitis
    (1)   Acute bronchitis
         (a)   Generally follows a viral respiratory infection
         (b)   May be caused by any number of respiratory viruses
         (c)   Symptoms include:
               (i)   Cough, usually productive
               (ii)   Shortness of breath
               (iii)   Wheezing
               (iv)   Rales, rhonchi
               (v)   Sore throat
         (d)   Provide care
               (i)   Consider inhaled bronchiodilators to open constricted air passages
               (ii)   Consider antibiotics only if sputum color changes to yellow, gray, or green
               (iii)   Consider mucolytic agents to moisten secretions
               (iv)   Provide supportive measures
                  *   Rest
                  *   Increase humidity to soothe air passages
                  *   Increase fluid intake
                  *   Refer to MD/PA for treatment

Chronic Obstructive Pulmonary Disease (COPD)
    (1)   The term COPD identifies patients with emphysema and chronic bronchitis. Although emphysema and chronic bronchitis are diagnosed as treated as separate diseases, most patients with COPD have features of both conditions. Chronic bronchitis is characterized by an excess of bronchial secretions. Emphysema

is characterized by a destruction of air spaces with permanent airspace enlargement

(2)   Causes include:
- (a)   Smoking- the most common
- (b)   Pollution
- (ci)   Infection
- (d)   Allergies

(3)   Symptoms include:
- (a)   Excessive, chronic cough
- (b)   Sputum production
- (c)   Chronic, increasing shortness of breath
- (d)   Dyspnea on exertion (DOE)
- (e)   In early stages of the disease, patient may be asymptomatic

(4)   Provide care
- (a)   COPD is largely preventable. Stress smoking cessation
- (b)   Consider respiratory treatments to facilitate the removal of thick mucous from airways
- (c)   Suggest breathing exercises
- (d)   Vaccination against influenza and pneumococcal disease
- (e)   Refer patient to MD/PA for treatment

Pneumonia

(1)   Viral
- (a)   Inflammation of lungs caused by a viral infection
- (b)   Two most common viral infections that cause pneumonia
  - (i)   Respiratory syncytial virus - Pediatrics
  - (ii)   Influenza
- (c)   Symptoms include:
  - (i)   Cough
  - (ii)   Headache
  - (iii)   Muscle stiffness
  - (iv)   Shortness of breath
  - (v)   Fever
  - (vi)   Sweating
  - (vii) Fatigue
- (d)   Provide care - supportive care
  - (i)   Humidified air
  - (ii)   Increase fluids
  - (iii)   Supplemental oxygen may be indicated
  - (iv)   Antiviral medications may be considered. Consult MD/PA for treatment

(2)   Bacterial
- (a)   Inflammation of lungs caused by bacterial infection
- (b)   Caused by different organisms and can range in seriousness. Two common types of organisms are:
  - (i)   Pneumococcal
  - (ii)   Mycoplasma
- (c)   Symptoms include:

            (i)   Rigors
            (ii)   Bloody sputum
            (iii)   Fever
            (iv)   Chest pain

(d)   Provide care
            (i)   Treat with antibiotics as directed by MD/PA
            (ii)   Provide supportive treatment

(3)   Asthma

(a)   Chronic inflammatory disorder characterized by increasing responsiveness of the airways to multiple stimuli

            (i)   Most acute attacks are reversible and improve spontaneously or within minutes to hours with treatment

            (ii)   The recognition that asthma is a chronic inflammatory disorder of the airways has significant implications for diagnosis, management, and potential prevention

            (iii)   Asthma is common in adults and more common in children. Death rates from asthma have been increasing since 1990, despite improved therapies

(b)   Occur spontaneously or can be triggered by:
            (i)   Respiratory infections
            (ii)   Exercise
            (iii)   Cold air
            (iv)   Smoke and other pollutants
            (v)   Stress or anxiety
            (vi)   Allergies

(c)   Symptoms include:
            (i)   Tightness in chest
            (ii)   Audible expiratory wheeze
            (iii)   Tachypnea
            (iv)   Course breath sounds
            (v)   Prolonged expiration
            (vi)   Restlessness/anxiety
            (vii)   Paroxysmal cough progressing from dry and hacking to productive
            (viii)   Diaphoresis

(d)   Identify key historical points
            (i)   Pattern of symptoms
                *   Perennial
                *   Seasonal
                *   Perennial and seasonal
                *   Continual
                *   Episodic
                *   Onset
                *   Duration
                *   Frequency
             (ii)   Aggravating factors
             (iii)   History of disease

   * Age of onset and method of diagnosis
   * Course of disease
   * Present management and medications
   * History or oral corticosteroid use
   * Intensive care unit admissions
   * History of intubation for asthma exacerbation
   * Other medical diseases
  (iv) Family history
  (v) Social history
   * Condition of home
   * Exposure to allergens
   * Smoking
   * Identification of participating causes
  (vi) Medications used

(e) Identify risk factors
  (i) Past history of sudden severe exacerbations
  (ii) Prior intubation for asthma
  (iii) Prior admissions for asthma to an intensive care unit
  (iv) Two or more hospitalizations for asthma in past year
  (v) Three or more emergency care visits for asthma in past year
  (vi) Use of more than two canisters per month
  (vii) Current use of systemic Corticosteroids or recent withdrawal from systemic corticosteroids

(f) Provide care
  (i) Inhaled bronchodilators
  (ii) Inhaled corticosteroids
  (iii) Oral corticosteroids
  (iii) Supportive care
   * Nebulization with inhaled sympathomimetics
   * Monitor pulse oximetry
   * Monitor BP and pulse after each nebulization
  (iv) Yearly influenza vaccine
  (v) Pneumococcal vaccine
  (vi) Refer patient to MD/PA for treatment - medical emergency

(g) Status asthmaticus- Severe prolonged asthma refractory to conventional modes of therapy. Management consists of:
  (i) Oxygen therapy
  (ii) Nebulization with inhaled bronchodilators
  (iii) Intravenous corticosteroids
  (iv) Intravenous fluids
  (v) May progress to require endotracheal intubation and mechanical ventilation

Administer prescribed inhaler

    (1)   Reassess patient history

    (2)   If medication is not prescribed to that patient, gain permission from MD/PA or follow local SOP

    (3)   Administration

          (a)   Patient should first inhale deeply

          (b)   Have patient place lips around opening of inhaler

          (c)   Press inhaler to activate the spray as the patient inhales deeply

          (d)   Patient should hold their breath as long as possible to ensure medication is absorbed

    (4)   Verify effectiveness. Repeat second dose as needed and according to SOP or MD/PA

Administer prescribed inhaler

    (1)   Reassess patient history

    (2)   If medication is not prescribed to that patient, gain permission from MD/PA or follow local SOP

    (3)   Administration

          (a)   Patient should first inhale deeply

          (b)   Have patient place lips around opening of inhaler

          (c)   Press inhaler to activate the spray as the patient inhales deeply

          (d)   Patient should hold their breath as long as possible to ensure medication is absorbed

    (4)   Verify effectiveness. Repeat second dose as needed and according to SOP or MD/PA

TERMINAL LEARNING OBJECTIVE

Given a standard fully stocked M5 Bag or Combat Medic Vest System, IV administration equipment and fluids, oxygen, suction and ventilation equipment (if available), selected medications, and documentation forms, You encounter a casualty complaining of gastrointestinal symptoms. No other injury(ies) are present. Treat gastrointestinal symptoms IAW cited references.

General assessment

Take focused history for gastrointestinal symptoms

(1)   OPQRST
      (a)   O-Onset
      (b)   P-Provoking/palliative factors
      (c)   Q-Quality
      (d)   R-Region/Radiation
      (e)   S-Severity
      (f)   T-Time
(2)   Allergies
(3)   Medications
(4)   Past medical history/past surgical history
(5)   Previous history of similar events
(6)   Nausea/ vomiting
(7)   Change in bowel habits/ stool
      (a)   Constipation
      (b)   Diarrhea
(8)   Weight loss/ Appetite changes
(9)   Last meal
(10) Chest pain
(11) Urinary symptoms- burning on urination, frequency
(12) Fever, shakes, chills

Abdominal examination

Note: The abdomen is divided into four quadrants by imaginary lines crossing at the umbilicus — the Right Upper Quadrant (RUQ), Left Upper Quadrant (LUQ), Right Lower Quadrant (RLQ), and Left Lower Quadrant (LLQ)

(1)   Inspection: check for scars, bruising, rashes, dilated veins, umbilical hernia or abdominal distention (swelling)
(2)   Auscultation: listen for bowel sounds. An arterial bruit (a vascular murmur like sound) may be heard and is always abnormal. Bowel sounds may be present, hyperactive, or absent. If sounds are not heard in five minutes of continuous auscultation, consider them absent.
(3)   Percussion: begin to percuss the liver down from the right upper chest. Liver dullness begins around the 5th or 6th rib extending

down to the costal (rib) margin. Liver length is usually less than 15 cm.

(4)   Palpation: palpate superficially (lightly) and deeper in all quadrants with the patients knees bent to relax the abdominal wall muscles. Assess for tenderness in all 4 quadrants. (will add picture for students)

    (a)   RUQ: palpate for the liver during inspiration, usually not palpated. If enlarged, you will feel the edge of the liver as it passes beneath the fingers.

    (b)   LUQ: palpate for the spleen on inspiration, usually not palpable.

    (c)   RLQ and LLQ: palpate for tenderness (pain increased by pressure). Check for involuntary guarding (tightness of the abdomen), and for rebound tenderness by quickly releasing pressure from the abdomen. Check for peritoneal irritation using the heeltap test.

(5)   Rectal Exam: with the patient standing while bending at the waist or curled on his/her side and using a glove and lubricant, slowly insert your index finger. Check the prostate anteriorly (in males) and obtain a stool specimen for blood and test using the hemocult test. This may be outside the scope of 91W.

(6)   The Routine Abdominal Examination:

    (a)   Inspect abdomen

    (b)   Auscultate all four quadrants

    (c)   Percuss liver size

    (d)   Palpate for enlarged liver

    (e)   Rectal examination for blood in stool

    (f)   ALWAYS include cardiac and respiratory examination when performing an abdominal examination

    (g)   ALWAYS consider whether a male or female genital examination by a M.D./P.A. may be required for complete assessment for the patient. All patients with abdominal pain require genital exam.

Assess for abdominal pain

(1)   Types of abdominal pain

    (a)   Somatic pain – Sharp, localized pain that originates in the peritoneal walls. Often described as a stabbing or burning pain

    (b)   Visceral pain – Poorly localized pain that originates in the walls of hollow organs. Often described as a vague, dull or cramping pain

    (c)   Referred pain – is pain that is felt at a location removed from the diseased organ that is causing pain

Identify and manage specific gastrointestinal illness

Upper Gastrointestinal (GI) Disease

(1)   Gastroenteritis: an acute syndrome characterized by inflammation of the stomach and intestinal tract. Viral or bacterial infections are the most common cause of acute gastroenteritis

    (a)   Signs and symptoms

        (i)   Nausea, vomiting and diarrhea-may be mild or severe

        (ii)   Fever- may or may not be present

        (iii)   Abdominal cramping. Normal to increased bowel sounds

        (iv)   Rectal examination may show blood in the stool

        (v)   May become dehydrated if fluid loss is severe

    (b)   Treatment:

        (i)   Rest

        (ii)   Correct fluid loss- either orally or with IV hydration

        (iii)   If vomiting is severe, control with an antiemetic, either orally or by intravenous injection at direction of physician. Contraindicated with invasive organisms.

        (iv)   Refer to a MD/PA for further care, especially when fever, severe abdominal pain or rectal blood is present

(2)   Upper GI Bleeding

    (a)   The vomiting of blood (hematemesis), passage of black tarry stool (melena), or occult chronic bleeding from the GI tract

    (b)   Caused by a number of factors such as: cancerous tumors, peptic ulceration, erosive gastritis, and esophageal varices

    (c)   Signs and symptoms: the manifestations of GI bleeding depend on the source, rate of bleeding, and underlying or coexistent disease. Patients with chronic blood loss may present with symptoms and signs of anemia (e.g., weakness, easy fatigability, pallor, chest pain, and dizziness) or chronic rectal bleeding.

    (d)   Treatment

        (i)   Hematemesis or melena is a medical emergency

        (ii)   Fluid resuscitation and treatment for shock are indicated

        (iii)   Refer to a PA/MD for more definitive care

        (iv)   Evacuate as soon as possible

(3)   Peptic Ulcer Disease: erosion of the lining of the stomach or duodenum as a result of gastric acid hyperacidity

    (a)   Risk factors- stress, diet, alcohol, caffeine, drugs (ASA, NSAIDs), tobacco, H. Pylori infection and heredity

    (b)   Signs and symptoms

        (i)   Epigastric pain 45-60 minutes after a meal

        (ii)   May be nocturnal — becoming most severe between midnight and 0200 hrs.

        (iii)   Pain, described as burning, may be relieved by food or antacid intake

        (iv)   Epigastric tenderness, occult blood on rectal exam if the ulcer is bleeding

        (v)   UGI or endoscopy confirms the diagnosis

  (c)   Treatment

        (i)   Restriction of coffee, tea, cola, alcohol, aspirin, NSAIDs and tobacco

        (ii)   Antacids: 30 ml P.O. 1 and 3 hours after meals and at bedtime, Cimetidine (Tagamet) 400 mg P.O. BID or 800 mg P.O. at bedtime.

        (iii)   Refer to MD/PA for full evaluation

(4)   Esophageal varices: An esophageal varix is a dialated vein of the esophagus. Primary causes of esophageal varices are alcohol consumption, portal hypertension, and the ingestion of caustic substances.

  (a)   Signs and symptoms: the physical findings in esophageal varices are:

        (i)   Hematemesis with bright red blood

        (ii)   Dysphagia (difficulty swallowing)

        (iii)   Burning or tearing sensation as the varices continue to bleed, irritating the lining of the esophagus

        (iv)   May exhibit classic signs of shock, including tachycardia, tachypnea and cool diaphoretic skin

  (b)   Treatment:

        (i)   Two large bore IV's

        (ii)   Treatment for shock and immediate evacuation to a definitive care facility

(5)   Esophageal reflux: "Gastroesophageal Reflux Disease" (GERD) is a term applied to the symptoms of tissue damage caused by the reflux of gastric contents (usually acidic) into the esophagus

  (a)   Signs and symptoms

        (i)   Heartburn, burping, regurgitation — worse when lying down, frequently severe substernal pain, occurring 30 — 60 minutes after eating

        (ii)   May manifest as laryngitis, chronic cough due to aspiration of gastric contents

        (iii)   The physical exam is usually normal

        (iv)   Cardiac disease MUST be ruled out prior to a diagnosis of reflux esophagitis is given

  (b)   Treatment:

        (i)   Weight reduction if obese

        (ii)   Avoid eating near bedtime

        (iii)   Antacids after meals and at bedtime

        (iv)   Avoid tobacco, alcohol and caffeine

(v)   Elevation of the head of the bed with 6 inch blocks helps

(vi)   Avoid large meals

(vii)   Tagament, Zantac, and Prilosec are oral medications to be used to reduce acid reflux

Lower Gastrointestinal (GI) Disease

(1)   Constipation: considered if defecation is delayed for days beyond the patients normal, or if the stools are unusually hard, dry, and difficult to move

     (a)   Signs and symptoms: difficulty or straining on defecation, occasionally with abdominal cramping. Usually no severe pain, nausea, vomiting or blood in stools. Normal bowel sounds on physical examination. Usually has no bleeding on hemoccult rectal exam.

     (b)   Treatment: increase intake of water and fiber (fruits, bulky vegetables, and bran cereals. Daily exercise. Metamucil 2 tsp. in water or juice 2 —3 x qd Milk of Magnesia 2 tsp. at Hs Bisacodyl (Dulcolax) 10 — 15 mg orally or suppository one rectally at hs, Fleets enemas.

(2)   Diarrhea: frequent passage of unformed watery bowel movements. May be due to viral, bacterial or parasitic infections

     (a)   Four basic mechanisms of diarrhea

         (i)   Increased intestinal secretion

         (ii)   Decreased intestinal absorption

         (iii)   Increased osmotic load

         (iv)   Abnormal intestinal motility

     (b)   Signs and symptoms

         (i)   Frequent, loose or watery stools

         (ii)   Change in consistency

         (iii)   Bloody (refer to Colitis) or nonbloody

         (iv)   Mucus

         (v)   Pus

         (vi)   Fatty materials, oil, grease (stools will float if high in fat)

         (vii)   Character and volume

             *   Describe the stools appearance: watery, bloody, or black and tar-like?

             *   How long does it last? Number of bowel movements per day?

             *   Do you have cramping associated with the bowel movement

     (c)   Etiology

         (i)   Can be caused by nerves, viral, or bacterial infection

         (ii)   Nocturnal diarrhea may suggest organic disease of the bowel

         (iii)   Toxic substances

         (iv)   May be found in family history of GI disorders

(v)	Different food or water as in history of travel
(vi)	Poor water or food sanitation or poor hygiene (Food Poisoning)
(vii)	Sexual transmission
(viii)	May have fever associated with dehydration
(ix)	Determine circumstances surrounding the onset

* **Acute diarrhea** - usually caused by infection; chronic may be caused by systemic illness; intermittent by psychological factors: Did it begin rapidly or gradually?; Were you under any stress at the time of onset?;
  What foods did you eat before it began?; Have you recently changed your diet?; Any travel history? Camping? Deployment?
* **Chronic**: when do you last recall not having the symptom?
* **Intermittent**: How long do intervals between episodes last?; Does diarrhea alternate with constipation?

(d) Treatment

(i)	Dictated by cause when known
(ii)	Clear liquids for 24 hours, then diet as tolerated

* Replacing lost fluid and electrolytes is the most important therapeutic measure in acute diarrhea
* If patient is significantly dehydrated, start IV fluid
* If patient is not vomiting and mild dehydration: oral rehydration

(iii)	Avoidance of agents that worsen diarrhea:

* Caffeine
* Dairy products
* Raw fruits and vegetables

(iv)	Kaopectate indicated only if illness and diarrhea continues
(v)	May give Lomotil or Imodium if no blood in stool or no fever
(vi)	If febrile or blood in stool, refer to MD/PA for antibiotic therapy and lab studies
(vii)	Withhold food for 24 hrs — clear liquid diet only, force clear liquids. Kaopectate liquid: 2 tbs. after each loose bowel movement (or 2 tbs.). Refer to MD/PA if not improved.

(3) Lower GI Bleeding

(a)	Signs and symptoms: Hematochezia (passage of bright red rectal blood), melena (dark or black tarry stool). 10% of hematochezia is due to an UGI bleed (Fast transit of blood)

(b)   Caused by a number of factors: colitis, malignancy, anorectal disease, inflammatory bowel disease, hemorroids

(c)   Treatment

     (i)   Hematochezia and melena are medical emergencies

     (ii)   Initiate two Large Bore IV's

     (iii)   Fluid resuscitation and treatment for shock are indicated

     (iv)   Referral to an MD/PA for definitive management

     (v)   Evacuate as soon as possible

(4)   Colitis: the term colitis applies to inflammatory diseases of the colon (e.g. ulcerative, granulomatous, ischemic, radiation, infectious colitis or irritable bowel syndrome)

     (a)   Signs and symptoms: bloody diarrhea of varied intensity and duration is interspersed with asymptomatic intervals. Usually an attack begins insidiously, with increased urgency to defecate, mild lower abdominal cramps, and blood and mucus in the stools. However, an attack may be acute and fulminant, with sudden violent diarrhea, high fever, signs of peritonitis, and profound toxemia. Some cases develop following a documented infection (e.g., amebiasis, bacillary dysentery).

     (b)   Treatment: dependent on diagnosis. Initial onset to be considered a medical emergency. Refer to MD/PA for management

(5)   Appendicitis: obstruction of the appendix by a fecalith, inflammation, foreign body or tumor

     (a)   Signs

          (i)   Classic presentation: Anorexia and pain in the epigastric or periumbilical area of the abdomen that evolves into pain in RLQ over 8 hours, often, signs and symptoms do not follow classic presentation

          (ii)   Nausea, diarrhea, and vomiting may accompany pain. Occasionally, constipation is present. The pain is moderately severe and after several hours localizes to the RLQ

          (iii)   Acute abdomen

          (iv)   Patient often will point precisely to the RLQ area of pain (positive McBurney's sign)

     (b)   Symptoms

          (i)   Abdominal tenderness

          (ii)   Fever may be present

          (iii)   Decreased bowel sounds if perforated

          (iv)   Rebound tenderness

          (v)   Rovsing sign (peritoneal irritation producing right lower quadrant pain with palpation of the left lower quadrant)

        (vi)   Psoas sign (pain with active flexion against resistance or passive extension of the right hip)

        (vii)   Obturator sign (pain with passive internal rotation of the flexed right hip)

        (viii)   Voluntary or involuntary guarding

        (ix)   Rectal tenderness is common

    (c)   Treatment: Appendicitis is a surgical emergency. Refer to PA/MD and evacuate immediately

(6)   Diverticular Disease: typically presents with left lower quadrant pain and tenderness, similar to the right-sided pain and tenderness of appendicitis

    (a)   Signs and symptoms:

        (i)   Abdominal pain, usually in the left lower quadrant

        (ii)   Nausea and vomiting

        (iii)   Constipation

        (iv)   Diarrhea

        (v)   Left lower quadrant tenderness, guarding, rebound

        (vi)   Fever

        (vii)   General peritonitis with tachycardia, high fever, and sepsis if colonic perforation occurs

    (b)   Treatment

        (i)   Diverticular disease is primarily a clinical diagnosis

        (ii)   Outpatient treatment: bowel rest and broad-spectrum oral antibiotic therapy. Patients are instructed to limit activity and maintain a liquid diet for 48 hours. If symptoms improve, low-residue foods are added to the diet.

        (iii)   If patient demonstrates signs of toxicity: fever, tachycardia, leukocytosis and severe abdominal pain, intravenous antibiotics are administered (authorized by MD/PA)

(7)   Bowel Obstruction: complete arrest or serious impairment of the passage of intestinal contents caused by a mechanical blockage. Mechanical obstruction is divided into obstruction of the small bowel, including the duodenum, and the large bowel. Major causes are hernia and adhesions

    (a)   Signs and symptoms:

        (i)   Obstruction of the small bowel is based on a triad of symptoms:

                *   Abdominal cramps are centered around the umbilicus or in the epigastrium; if cramps become severe and steady, consider strangulation (lack of blood flow to the bowel)

                *   Vomiting starts early with small-bowel and late with large-bowel obstruction

          *   Constipation occurs with complete obstruction, but diarrhea may be present with partial obstruction

    (ii)   Obstruction of the large bowel: symptoms usually develop more gradually than with small-bowel obstruction. Increasing constipation leads to obstipation and abdominal distention. If the ileocecal valve is competent, there may be no vomiting; if it allows reflux of colonic contents into the ileum, vomiting may occur (usually several hours after onset of symptoms). Lower abdominal cramps unproductive of feces are present.

(b)   Treatment

    (i)   A nasogastric tube is inserted and placed on suction

    (ii)   An inlying bladder catheter helps monitor urinary output

    (iii)   IV hydration

    (iv)   Complete obstruction is treated surgically after supportive therapy has been initiated

    (v)   Bowel obstruction should be considered a surgical emergency. Refer patient to an MD/PA and evacuate immediately

(7)   Hemorrhoids: a varicose vein in the lower rectum or anus. Caused by straining at stool, constipation, prolonged sitting and a diet poor in fiber.

    (a)   Signs and symptoms: itching, irritation and bleeding with bowel movements. Obvious external hemorrhoid or internal hemorrhoids found on rectal examination. Mucoid discharge from rectum

    (b)   Treatment: high roughage/fiber diet. Sitz bath (sitting in warm water reduces pain and swelling). Metamucil 2 tsp. in water or juice 1-3 times daily. Anusol or Anusol HC suppositories for internal hemorrhoids can be given two-three times a day.

    (c)   Complications: A thrombosed hemorrhoid is caused by the rupture of a vein, forming a clot in the subcutaneous tissue. A tender bluish mass is visualized. Thrombosed hemorrhoids require evaluation by an MD/PA.

Liver, Biliary Tract and Pancreatic Diseases

(1)   Hepatitis

    (a)   Hepatitis is a liver inflammation that stems from a virus or hepatotoxic agent

    (b)   Viral hepatitis is the most common of the serious, contagious diseases caused by a virus that attacks the liver

(c)   Hepatitis B & C are classified as sexually transmitted diseases

(d)   Types

      (i)   Hepatitis A - formerly called infectious hepatitis
* Ranks as most common type of hepatitis
* Highly contagious
* Transmitted primarily in food handled by individuals in the infectious stages of the disease is very contagious and often spread within families
* Public health problems occur from contaminated shellfish after raw sewage releases and accidents as well as, from commercial food handlers
* Acute onset
* No treatment has been shown to alter the disease course
* Immunization: An inactivated hepatitis A vaccine is available, Prophylactic IG may be administered within two weeks after exposure to hepatitis A, Persons traveling to Africa, the Middle East, Central and South America, and Asia should be immunized FEMA team personnel should be offered vaccine if they travel out of the United States

      (ii)   Hepatitis B - formerly called serum hepatitis; most serious form
* A prominent source of acute/chronic hepatitis and cirrhosis of the liver
* Hepatitis B virus is very hardy, the virus' ability to survive outside its normal environment for an extended period of time demonstrates the need for appropriate application of universal precautions
* Signs and symptoms are vague and can be mistaken for influenza or the common cold (fatigue, gastrointestinal disorders, headaches)
* In prehospital care workers, needle stick injuries, mucous membrane contact and open lesions of the skin are the primary mode
* Needle stick injuries are the most common cause of contraction

     *   Workers are at risk of HBV infection to the extent they are exposed to blood and body fluids

     *   Modes of transmission are preventable by the application of engineering controls, proper work practices (universal precautions), and HBV vaccination

     *   Prophylaxis: Hepatitis B vaccine before exposure and Hepatitis B immune globulin after exposure

   (iii)   Hepatitis C - formerly called non A, non B hepatitis

     *   Transmission: transfused blood (most common), body fluids

     *   Individuals at high risk for developing hepatitis C include: Intravenous drug users, renal dialysis patients, multi-transfused patients, hemophiliacs

     *   Prevention: clean water supply, safe disposal of human waste, hygienic handling of food, good personal hygiene, and medical prophylaxis includes active immunization with Immunoglobulin (1g)

     *   Treatment: no specific treatment or drug can kill the hepatitis viruses

(3)   Acute pancreatitis: inflammation of the pancreas- alcoholism accounts for 80% of all causes

  (a)   Signs and symptoms

     (i)   Abrupt onset of epigastric pain, radiating to back

     (ii)   Nausea, vomiting, sweating, weakness

     (iii)   Abdominal tenderness and distention

     (iv)   Fever

     (v)   May have a history of previous episodes, often related to alcohol abuse

     (vi)   Jaundice may occur – may be caused by stones

  (b)   Treatment:

     (i)   NPO until patient is pain free

     (ii)   Nasogastric suction

     (iii)   IV hydration

     (iv)   Bed rest

     (v)   Pain control with narcotics IV (by MD/PA order)

     (vi)   Refer patient to MD/PA

     (vii)   Evacuate as soon as possible

(4)   Acute Cholecystitis: acute inflammation of the gallbladder wall, usually as a response to cystic duct obstruction by a gallstone

  (a)   Signs and symptoms

           (i)   Steady, severe pain and tenderness in the right upper quadrant or umbilical area. Acute attack is often precipitated by a large, fatty meal.

           (ii)   Nausea and vomiting

           (iii)   Painful splinting of respiration during deep inspiration and right upper quadrant palpation (Murphy's sign) is frequent

           (iv)   Fever

      (b)   Treatment

           (i)   NPO

           (ii)   IV hydration

           (iii)   Pain control with narcotics IV (by MD/PA order)

           (iv)   IV antibiotics – as directed by MD/PA

           (v)   Cholecystectomy usually performed 2-3 days after acute episode subsides

           (vi)   Refer patient to MD/PA

           (vii)   Evacuate as soon as possible

(5)   Cholelithiasis: formation or presence of calculi (gallstones) in the gallbladder.

      (a)   Signs and symptoms

           (i)   The clinical consequences of stone formation in the gallbladder are exceedingly variable. Most patients remain asymptomatic for long periods, frequently for life.

           (ii)   Persistent obstruction usually produces inflammation and acute cholecystitis. Stones in the duct cause colicky pain associated with peristaltic motion.

      (b)   Treatment: symptomatic gallstones - biliary colic recurs with irregular, pain-free intervals of days or months. Symptomatic patients are at increased risk of developing complications, and cholecystectomy is indicated. Refer to PA/MD and evacuate.

TERMINAL LEARNING OBJECTIVE

Given a standard fully stocked M5 Bag or Combat Medic Vest System, IV administration equipment and fluids, oxygen, suction, and ventilation equipment (if available), selected medications, and documentation forms. You encounter a casualty complaining of genitourinary problems. No other injury(ies) are present. Performed initial management interventions for genitourinary symptoms identified during focus history and exam.

Recognize specific illnesses

Cystitis

(1)   Definition - inflammation of the urinary bladder

Urine is normally sterile. Bacteria reach the bladder by way of infected kidneys, lymphatics, and the urethra. Because the urethra is short in women, ascending infections are more common in women.

(2)   Causes
- (a)   Fecal contamination
- (b)   Catheters
- (c)   Sexual intercourse - occurs after long periods without sexual intercourse. Also called "Honeymoon cystitis"

(3)   Symptoms
- (a)   Urgency (a feeling of the need to void although the bladder is not full)
- (b)   Frequency
- (c)   Dysuria (painful urination)
- (d)   Perineal and suprapubic pain
- (e)   Hematuria
- (f)   Chills and fever are rare, but may indicate a more serious illness

(4)   Diagnosis
- (a)   Patient's history and physical examination
- (a)   Urinalysis, urine culture and sensitivity (C&S)—may show an increase in the number of red and white cells, as well as the causative microorganism

(5)   Treatment
- (a)   Increase fluid intake
- (b)   Identify and correct contributing factors
- (c)   Antimicrobial therapy as prescribed by the MD/PA
- (d)   Urinary (Pyridium) for dysuria

Urethritis

(1)   Definition - inflammation of the urethra, more common in men than in women

(2)   Causes
- (a)   If caused by organisms other than gonorrhea--it is known as nonspecific urethritis (NSU)

      (b)   Gonorrhea causes a specific form of infection that can attack the mucous membrane of the urethra

      (c)   Urethritis may accompany cystitis in women

      (d)   Nonspecific urethritis in men caused by:

            (i)   Irritation during vigorous intercourse

            (ii)   Intercourse with an infected partner

            (iii)   Most common cause of urethritis is caused by chlamydia trachomatis

(3)   Symptoms

      (a)   Dysuria - ranging from slight tickling to burning or severe discomfort

      (b)   Urinary frequency

      (c)   Fever is NOT common and implies a more serious infection to prostate, testes, and epididymis in males

      (d)   Urethral discharge

(4)   Diagnosis

      (a)   Patient's history and symptoms

      (b)   In men, urethral smear (gram stain)/ C & S to identify causative organism

      (c)   In women, clean catch urinalysis

(5)   Treatment

      (a)   Antibiotic therapy as prescribed by the MD/PA. Depending on organism must involve MD/PA as treatment needs to be tailored and treatment of syphilis is also required in many cases.

      (b)   Increase fluid intake

      (c)   Analgesics for pain/discomfort

Pyelonephritis

(1)   Definition - infection of the renal parenchyma (the functional tissue of an organ as distinguished from supporting or connective tissue) and the lining of the collecting system

(2)   Causes

      (a)   Acute pyelonephritis

            (i)   Associated with diabetes, pregnancy and extremes of age

            (ii)   Bacterial infection such as E-coli, streptococcus, pseudomonas, and staph aureus

            (iii)   More common causes are bladder instrumentation, neurogenic bladder, and inability to completely empty the bladder

      (b)   Risk factors

            (i)   Diabetes

            (ii)   Pregnancy

            (iii)   Recent instrumentation

            (iv)   Extremes of age

(3)   Symptoms

      (a)   Acute pyelonephritis

            (i)   Flank pain

          (ii)   Chills, fever, and malaise
          (iii)   Frequency and burning on urination may be
                     present if bladder is also infected.
          (iv)   Nausea and vomiting, dehydration with
                     secondary
          (v)   Headache

(4)   Diagnosis
          (a)   Urinalysis positive for leukocyte (WBC's) casts
          (b)   Positive urine culture
          (c)   Physical examination reveals CVA (costovertebral angle)
                     or flank tenderness

(5)   Treatment
          (a)   Symptomatic treatment for fever and pain
          (b)   Antibiotic therapy prescribed by MD/PA. May consider
                     ampicillin. gentamycin or fluoroquinolone (Cipro/Levaquin)
          (c)   Liberal oral fluid intake, if unable to tolerate fluids IV
                     hydration and antibiotics
          (d)   Relief of any urinary obstruction
          (e)   All patients need to be evaluated by a physician

NOTE: Damage to the kidney can be life threatening if not treated promptly.

(6)   Discharge Teaching
          (a)   Follow diet and fluid regime as prescribed
          (b)   Take medications exactly as directed
                 (i)   Do not omit or discontinue medication unless
                         told by the physician
                 (ii)   Do not take nonprescription drugs unless
                         cleared by the physician

Infections of the female reproductive system

(1)   Vaginitis
          (a)   Definition - inflammation of the vagina (The normal acidity
                     of the vaginal secretion is a natural defense against
                     infection but, if infected by certain pathogenic organisms,
                     an infection results)
          (b)   Causes
                 (i)   Bacteria- most common
                 (ii)   Trichomonas vaginalis - a protozoan
                 (iii)   Candida albicans – yeast (fungal)
          (c)   Facts
                 (i)   Commonly occurs during pregnancy and after
                         antibiotic therapy
                 (ii)   Frequently seen in women with diabetes
                 (iii)   Vaginitis may persist for years
                 (iv)   Factors that influence the development of a
                         vaginal infection include
                     *   A change in the vaginal ph.

        *   Hormonal changes during the menstrual cycle, pregnancy or for any other reason (such as taking steroids).

        *   Long-term use of birth control pills

        *   Use of systemic antibiotics

        *   Compromised immunity

(d)   Types of Vaginitis:

    (i)   Bacterial Vaginosis (BV)

        *   Known as nonspecific vaginitis.

        *   Caused by a combination of organisms.

        *   Increased discharge (white, yellow or gray) with a "fishy" odor.

        *   Redness or edema not significant.

        *   May be sexually transmitted

    (ii)   Trichomonas Vaginalis (Trichomoniasis) - a sexually transmitted disease

    (iii)   Candidiasis albicans— "typical yeast infection" may be a sexually transmitted disease

(e)   Signs and symptoms

    (i)   Leukorrhea - whitish or yellow white vaginal discharge

    (ii)   Discharge may be frothy or thick

    (iii)   Odorous and profuse discharge (more so in trichomoniasis)

    (iv)   Perineal, vaginal and urethral burning and itching

    (v)   Possible discomfort in lower abdominal region

    (vi)   Redness or rash around vagina

    (vii)   Painful intercourse

    (viii) Occasionally asymptomatic

NOTE: Diagnosis is made upon microscopic examination of the vaginal discharge (usually a wet prep/KOH) and normal saline.

    (f)   Treatment

      (i)   Metronidazole (Flagyl) if BV or trichomoniasis infection - dose 250mg po tid x7 days or 2gm po in single dose. Instruct patient not to drink alcohol while taking Flagyl and for three days after completion of therapy. Using together will cause nausea, vomiting, headache, cramps and flushing)

      (ii)   Nystatin cream (Mycostatin, Nilstat); Miconazole (Monistat, Micatin) Clotrimazole (Mycelex) if candida infection

      (iii)   If has glycosuria (glucose in urine), patient will need work-up to rule out the diagnosis of diabetes mellitus

        (iv)   Women with any of the following clinical situations should notify the physician at the first sign of a vaginal infection
* First vaginal infection
* Unsure if it is a yeast infection
* High risk for HIV or AIDS
* Diabetic
* Temperature over 100 degrees
* Under 12 years of age
* Pregnant
* New onset pain especially lower abdomen, back, or shoulder
* Malodorous vaginal discharge

(2)   Pelvic Inflammatory Disease (PID)

    (a)   Definition - an infection or inflammation of the ovaries, fallopian tubes, uterus, or pelvic cavity

    (b)   Causes and transmission
        (i)   Infection usually enters the pelvic organs (uterus fallopian tubes, ovaries) through the cervix and vagina
        (ii)   Organisms commonly associated with causing PID are N. gonorrhea and Chlamydia

    (c)   Signs and symptoms
        (i)   Foul-smelling vaginal discharge
        (ii)   Back ache
        (iii)   Pelvic pain
        (iv)   Abdominal pain
        (v)   Fever, chills, malaise
        (vi)   Nausea, vomiting
        (vii)   Menorrhagia
        (viii) Dysmenorrhea
        (ix)   Dyspareunia

    (d)   Risk factors
        (i)   Multiple sexual partners
        (ii)   History of STDs in the past
        (iii)   Frequent vaginal douching
        (iv)   IUD (intrauterine device for contraception)-highest risk first four months after insertion
        (v)   Younger age

    (e)   Diagnosis
        (i)   Based on symptoms and physical exam findings-lower abdominal pain is the most frequent presenting complaint
        (ii)   Wet prep (saline/KOH (potassium hydroxide) of vaginal secretions)
        (iii)   Culture and sensitivity of vaginal discharge to determine causative organism
        (iv)   Ultrasound if available
        (v)   This is a cause of serious illness and death if not treated quickly and properly – Patient may

> develop toxic shock syndrome that can be rapidly fatal.

(f) Treatment

    (i) Serious illness that requires hospitalization for administration of IV antibiotics and supportive care Patient must be treated quickly and properly.

    (ii) IV antibiotics as prescribed by the MD/PA

    (iii) During the active disease process, douches and sexual intercourse should be avoided

    (iv) Remove IUD if in place

(g) Discharge Teaching:

    (i) Both sex partners must be instructed to take their prescribed medications even though one partner may be asymptomatic

Kidney Stones

(1) Stones form throughout the urinary system. Patients usually present when the stone has migrated into a ureter

(2) Cause

    (a) Dehydration

    (b) Increase in minerals in water supply

    (c) Occurs three times more often in males than females

(3) Symptoms

    (a) Acute onset of severe flank pain

    (b) Flank pain radiates to the groin, scrotum or labia

    (c) Nausea, vomiting, secondary dehydration, anxious

    (d) Cool clammy skin, diaphoresis, tachycardia and increased blood pressure due to severe pain

    (e) Hematuria with dysuria, urinary frequency

(4) Diagnosis

    (a) Urine analysis – hematuria

    (b) Physical assessment - acute CVA /flank tenderness on affected side

    (c) Fever and/or hypotension are unusual and would suggest possibility of infection or diagnosis other than renal colic

(5) Differential Diagnosis

    (a) Aortic dissection

    (b) Abdominal aortic aneurysm

    (c) Renal obstruction

    (d) Acute myocardial infarction

    (e) Acute abdomen

(6) Treatment

    (a) Pain control-IV narcotics almost always required

    (b) IV hydration

    (c) Strain all urine to recover stone, if passed

    (d) Refer immediately to nearest MTF for management

Acute scrotal pain

(1)   Differential Diagnosis
        (a)   Testicular torsion
                (i)   Cause
                        *   History of athletic event or trauma
                (ii)   Symptoms
                        *   Pain is sudden and severe with
                             radiation into abdomen
                (iii)   Diagnosis
                        *   Malpositioned testes-lateral
                             orientation and elevated
                        *   Ultrasound
                (vi)   Treatment
                        *   Immediate referral to the nearest
                             treatment facility
                        *   Manual detorsion of the affected testis
                             may be attempted. This is
                             accomplished standing at the foot of
                             or on the right side of the patient's
                             bed. The torsed testis is detorsed in a
                             fashion similar to "opening a book".
                             That is, the patient's right testis is
                             rotated in a counterclockwise fashion
                             and the patient's left testis in a
                             clockwise fashion.
                        *   Surgical Emergency – patient will lose
                             testicle if torsion is not corrected
        (b)   Epididymitis
                (i)   Cause
                        *   Bacterial infection, often STD
                        *   Urinary tract infection
                        *   Prostatitis
                        *   Prolonged use of indwelling catheters
                (ii)   Signs and symptoms
                        *   Pain more gradual than onset of
                             torsion
                        *   Causes lower abdominal, inguinal and
                             scrotal or testicular pain alone or in
                             combination
                (iii)   Diagnosis
                        *   Painful urination
                        *   Transient relief of scrotal/testicular
                             pain In the recumbent position with
                             scrotal elevation
                        *   Pyuria (WBC's and bacteria) on
                             urinalysis
                        *   Epididymis tender on palpation. May
                             feel like a 'bag of worms"
                (iv)   Management

*	Antibiotic therapy as prescribed by MD/PA
*	Increase fluid intake – oral or IV
*	Rest with scrotal elevation
*	Oral analgesics

Sexual Assault Assessment

(1)   5% of violent crimes in U.S.
        (a)   Much higher incidence in 3rd world countries
        (b)   Grossly under reported
(2)   Assessment
        (a)   Assess for and treat any life-threatening injuries (compromised airway, hypovolemic shock)
        (b)   Provide "safe" environment –shield from other patients, visitors
        (c)   Avoid touching patient without permission
        (d)   Tell patient not to shower, bathe, change clothes or throw clothes away until examined by the physician. Evidence preservation is paramount.
        (e)   Notify MD/PA immediately

Recognize Sexually Transmitted Diseases

Factors that contribute to Sexually Transmitted Diseases (STD)

(1)   Unknown carrier of disease
(2)   Casual sex
(3)   Absence of laws that require reporting of ALL STDs
(4)   Length of time between exposure and appearance of symptoms (or positive antibody tests)
(5)   Failure to:
        (a)   Recognize signs and symptoms
        (b)   Seek early treatment
        (c)   Refrain from sexual activity until treatment complete
(6)   Lack of knowledge regarding STDs and their prevention
(7)   Failure of sexually active person to heed STD warnings

Factors related to prevention and control of STDs

(1)   Public education:
        (a)   School Systems
        (b)   Television and newspapers
(2)   Refrain from sexual activity until disease eradicated
(3)   Locate and treat contacts
(4)   Continued research
(5)   STD clinics

Chlamydia (Appears 7-10 Days after exposure)

(1)   Caused by the organism, Chlamydia trachomatis (parasite)
(2)   Signs and Symptoms
    (a)   Urethritis & epididymitis in men
    (b)   Cervicitis & macopurulent discharge in women
    (c)   Some patients may be asymptomatic, especially women
    (d)   Can be transmitted from mother to infant at birth
    (e)   Additional problems
        (i)   Pelvic inflammatory disease
        (ii)   Ectopic pregnancy
        (iii)   Sterility
        (iv)   Systemic infections
(3)   Diagnosis
    (a)   Direct microscopic examination-will observe flagellated parasite
    (b)   Culture of secretions or tissue scrapings
(4)   Management
    (a)   Antimicrobials, such as tetracycline, erythromycin, sulfonamide as prescribed by MD/PA
    (b)   Explain the prescribed treatment
        (i)   Length of treatment is 7-21 days
        (ii)   Patient should refrain from sexual activity during treatment
    (c)   Referral to Preventative Medicine for reporting

NOTE: Treatment failure can be due to either reinfection or patient noncompliance with antimicrobial therapy.

Gonorrhea

(1)   Caused by the organism Neisseria gonorrhea. Often co-exists with chlamydial infections.
(2)   Signs and Symptoms
    (a)   Appear 2 to 6 days after exposure
    (b)   Men
        (i)   Urethritis with a purulent discharge.
        (ii)   Pain on urination
        (iii)   May spread to prostate, seminal vesicles, epididymis
        (iv)   Sometimes there are no symptoms in men
        (v)   Gonococcal infection occur in the pharynx and rectum
    (c)   Women
        (i)   Vaginal discharge
        (ii)   Abnormal menstrual bleeding
        (iii)   Painful urination
        (iv)   80% experience no symptoms
(3)   Diagnosis
    (a)   Gram stain and culture

<table>
<tr><td>(b)</td><td>In men, specimen of urethral discharge is obtained; anal and pharyngeal smears if person has practiced anal or oral sex.</td></tr>
<tr><td>(c)</td><td>In women, specimen obtained from cervix</td></tr>
</table>

NOTE: Lubricants are not used on speculum because these products may destroy the gonococci.

(4)   Management
     (a)   Antibiotics as prescribed by MD/PA. Rocephin 250 mg IM is usually effective treatment
     (b)   Explain the treatment regimen
     (c)   Explain the importance of contacting all sexual partners for examination and treatment
     (d)   Refrain from sexual activity until follow-up smears are negative
     (e)   Referral to Preventative Medicine for reporting

Syphilis

(1)   Caused by spirochete, Treponema pallidum. If untreated, progresses through secondary & tertiary stages.

(2)   Signs and Symptoms
     (a)   Primary (early) stage (Appears 2-6 weeks after exposure)
         (i)   Chancre appears on genitals, anus, cervix, and other parts of body.
         (ii)   Chancre first resembles papule, later appears ulcerated, _painless_
         (iii)   Heals by itself in several weeks
     (b)   Secondary Stage: (Appears 2-6 weeks after primary stage)
         (i)   Fever
         (ii)   Malaise
         (iii)   Rash – most common manifestation
         (iv)   Headache
         (v)   Sore throat
         (vi)   Enlarged lymph nodes
     (c)   Tertiary Stage: Non-infectious – involvement of the nervous and cardiovascular systems
         (i)   May occur years after initial infection. Sometimes as much as twenty years later.

(3)   Diagnosis
     (a)   Lab tests (serum)
         (i)   VDRL - Venereal Disease Research Laboratory
         (ii)   RPR - Rapid Plasma Reagent
         (iii)   Fluorescent treponemal antibody absorption test

(4)   Management
     (a)   Explain the treatment regimen
     (b)   Instruct the patient to avoid intercourse until permitted
     (c)   Primary and secondary stages
         (i)   Penicillin G - drug of choice

              (ii)   Tetracycline or erythromycin - if allergic to penicillin

              (iii)   Follow-up examination at 3,6, & 12 months

      (d)   Tertiary stage:

              (i)   Larger doses of penicillin G

              (ii)   Response is poor in patients with cardio-vascular syphilis

Herpes Genitalis

(1)   Caused by Herpes Simplex Virus

(2)   Signs and Symptoms

      (a)   Painful vesicular lesions on buttocks, penis, perineum, vulva, cervix, vagina (if transmitted by anal intercourse, lesions may appear in rectum and perianal area).

      (b)   Lesions may persist for several weeks

      (c)   Malaise

      (d)   Fever

      (e)   Chills

      (f)   Headache

      (g)   Reoccurrence in 60 – 90 % of patients

(3)   Diagnosis

      (a)   Examination of lesions-linear vesicles. Microscopic exam will show giant cells.

      (b)   Viral culture

(4)   Management

      (a)   Acyclovir (Zovirax) - oral, topical, intravenous

NOTE: Acyclovir may decrease the frequency and magnitude of reoccurrences.

      (b)   Analgesics for pain and discomfort

      (c)   If eye infection, use Vira-A, Herpes Liquafilm or Viroptic

      (d)   Instruct the patient to use a condom at all times if there is a periodic reoccurrence of the lesions

      (e)   Refrain from sexual intercourse or use a condom

      (f)   Pregnant women must inform the physician if they have a history of herpes. Delivery during an active outbreak can be fatal to the infant.

Genital Warts

(1)   Caused by human papilloma virus (HPV)

(2)   Signs and Symptoms

      (a)   Incubation period is normally 1-2 months, but may be longer

      (b)   Painless, soft, fleshy wart-like growths on the genitalia or cervix or in vagina

(3)   Diagnosis: visual examination

(4)   Management

(a)	No cure
(b)	RPR for syphilis
(c)	Treat with podophyllin, a topical solution that is left in place for 4-6 hours, and then washed off
(d)	Teach the patient to use a condom

NOTE: There appears to be an increased risk of cancer of the vulva, cervix, and vagina in women with genital warts.

Review Male and Female Catheterization

Urinary Catheterization

(1) Definition - Insertion of a catheter (tube for injecting or removing fluids) through the urethra into the bladder for the purpose of removing urine.

(2) Purposes of Urinary Catheterization
  (a) Relieve urinary retention
  (b) Obtain sterile urine specimen from female
  (c) Measure amount of residual urine in bladder (an amount greater than 50 ml is considered abnormal)
  (d) Empty bladder before, during, and after surgery
  (e) To obtain a urine specimen when a specimen cannot be obtained by any other means

(3) Urinary Catheter Sizes
  (a) The smaller the number, the smaller the catheter
  (b) No. 8 Fr and 10 Fr - used for children
  (c) No. 14 Fr and 16 Fr - used for female adult
  (d) No. 18 Fr, 20 Fr - usually used for male adult

NOTE: Larger size catheter used for male because it is stiffer, thus easier to push the distance of the male urethra.

Types of Urinary Catheters

(1) Intermittent catheter
  (a) Used to drain bladder for short periods (5-10 min)
  (b) Commonly used for self-catheterization by patients in the home environment (after proper amount of training)
  (c) Commonly used with spinal cord injury patients

(2) Indwelling/retention catheter
  (a) Continuous bladder drainage
  (b) Gradual decompression of over-distended bladder

NOTE: Do not remove more than 750cc to 1000cc of urine from the bladder at any one time. Gradual decompression will prevent bladder damage and shock.

  (c) Intermittent bladder drainage and irrigation
  (d) Drainage tube and collection device connected to this type of catheter

    (e) Most commonly used indwelling catheter is a Foley catheter

      (i)   Designed with balloon at distal tip which can be inflated with sterile water or saline

      (ii) Inflated balloon keeps catheter from slipping out of bladder

(3) Supra pubic catheter

    (a) Inserted into bladder through small incision above pubic area

    (b) Occasionally used for continuous drainage

Procedure for the insertion of Foley Catheter in the male and female patient

It is important to remember that the bladder normally is a sterile cavity and the external opening to the urethra can never be sterilized. Pathogens introduced into the bladder can ascend the ureters and lead to bladder and kidney infections.

(1) Gather all equipment - wash hands

    (a) Sterile catheterization kit

    (b) Flashlight or lamp

    (c) Urine collection bag

    (d) Velcro leg strap or anchoring tape

    (e) Disposal bag

    (f) Waterproof pad or chux

(2) Explain procedure to patient. He/she may experience a burning/pressure sensation as the catheter is inserted, and a feeling of needing to void, once catheter is in place

(3) Provide for adequate lighting

(4) Provide for privacy

(5) Position patient

    (a) Males - assist patient into supine position with thighs slightly apart. First place waterproof pad under patient's buttocks. Drape patient so only penis is exposed.

    (b) Females - assist patient to dorsal recumbent position with knees flexed and about 2 feet apart. Females may also be positioned in the Sim's or lateral position with upper leg flexed. Place waterproof pad under patient.

(6) Cleanse genital and perineal areas with soap and water. Rinse and dry. Wash hands.

(7) Open sterile catheterization tray and supplies, using sterile technique.

(8) Put on sterile gloves. Open sterile drape and place on patient's thighs. Place drape with opening over penis (males) or labia (females).

(9) Place catheter set on or next to patient's legs on sterile drape.

(10) For indwelling catheters, test catheter balloon:

    (a) Attach pre-filled irrigation syringe to injection port

    (b) Inject appropriate amount of fluid

        (c)   If balloon inflates properly, withdraw fluid and leave syringe attached to port

(11)   Pour antiseptic solution over cotton balls

(12)   Lubricate catheter for about 6 to 7 inches (males) or 1-2 inches (females)

(13)   Insertion of Catheter

        (a)   Males

              (i)   Lift penis with non-dominant hand, which is then considered contaminated.

              (ii)   Retract foreskin in uncircumcised male

              (iii)   Cleanse area at meatus with a cotton ball that is held with forceps

              (iv)   Use circular motion, moving from meatus toward base of penis. Repeat this three times

              (v)   Hold penis with slight upward tension and perpendicular to patient's body

              (vi)   Instruct patient to bear down as if voiding

              (vii)   With dominant hand, place drainage end of catheter into receptacle (if pre-attached to drainage bag, place bag close to sterile field)

              (viii)   Insert catheter tip into meatus

              (ix)   Advance tip 6 to 8 inches until urine flows

              (x)   Do not use force to introduce catheter

              (xi)   For slight resistance, ask patient to take a deep breath and rotate catheter slightly

              (xii)   Once urine drains, advance catheter another 1/2 to 1 inch

              (xiii)   Inflate the balloon with the pre-filled syringe

        (b)   Females

              (i)   With thumb and one finger of non-dominant hand, spread labia and identify meatus. Maintain separation of labia with one hand

              (ii)   Using antiseptic soaked cotton balls held with forceps, cleanse area from clitoris toward anus, using a different sterile cotton ball each time-first to the right of the urinary meatus, then to the left of the urinary meatus then down the center over the urinary meatus. Discard each cotton ball after one downward stroke.

              (iii)   With sterile gloved hand, place drainage end of catheter into receptacle. (If pre-attached to drainage bag, place bag close to sterile field)

              (iv)   Insert catheter tip into meatus 2 to 3 inches or until urine flows.

              (v)   Do not use force to push catheter through urethra into bladder

              (vi)   For slight resistance, ask patient to take a deep breath and rotate catheter gently as it reaches external sphincter.

	(vii)	Once urine drains, advance catheter 1/2 to 1 inch
	(viii)	Inflate the balloon with the prefilled syringe
(14)	Check to insure balloon is properly filled:	
	(a)	Tug gently on catheter to feel for resistance
	(b)	Attach catheter to drainage system if required

(15)   Secure catheter to upper thigh (males and females) or lower abdomen with penis directed toward patient's chest (males). Leave some slack in catheter to prevent tension.
(16)   Secure drainage bag below level of bladder. Check that tubing is not kinked and movement of side rails does not impede drainage.
(17)   Cleanse and dry perineal area
(18)   Remove equipment and make patient comfortable
(19)   Wash your hands
(20)   Document procedure in record

(a)	Type and size of catheter
(b)	Time of catheterization
(c)	Amount of urine removed
(d)	Description of urine
(e)	Client's reaction to procedure
(f)	Client's teaching and level of understanding

Removing a Retention Bladder Catheter

(1)   Assemble all equipment

(a)	10 cc syringe
(b)	Waterproof drape
(c)	Soap and water
(d)	Exam gloves
(e)	Privacy drape

(2)   Explain procedure to patient, and advise that he/she may feel a slight burning sensation during removal of the catheter and the first time or two that they void.
(3)   Provide for privacy and assist female patient to a dorsal recumbent position, or the male patient to a supine position.
(4)   Place waterproof drape under patient's buttocks and provide a drape for patient privacy.
(5)   Wash hands and don disposable gloves
(6)   Remove securing tape on catheter
(7)   Attach syringe to balloon valve and aspirate entire amount of water from balloon. Check size of balloon so you know how much to remove.
(8)   Encourage patient to take deep breath and relax while gently removing catheter per ward SOP. Wrap catheter in towel or disposable waterproof drape.
(9)   Clean the perineal area after the catheter is removed.
(10)   Remove gloves and wash hands
(11)   Reposition patient comfortably

(12)   Instruct patient to drink plenty of fluids, if appropriate. Record intake and output, and instruct patient regarding need to void into bedpan or urinal.

(13)   Inform patient that it may take a while for   bladder to reestablish voluntary control, and that an accident is not unusual.

(14)   Discard equipment and return it to appropriate area

(15)   Record procedure, including the following
- (a)   Time of procedure
- (b)   Description and amount of urine in drainage bag
- (c)   Record all patient teaching accomplished and patient's level of understanding

(16)   Record and report any unusual signs to the charge nurse. These include, but are not limited to:
- (a)   Discomfort
- (b)   Bleeding
- (c)   Change in vital signs (Increased pulse/decreased BP)
- (d)   Increase in temperature
- (e)   Strong odor

Care of the patient with an indwelling urinary catheter

(1)   Catheter care
- (a)   Wash hands before and after catheter care
- (b)   Clean perineal area and proximal third of catheter twice a day and after bowel movements. Use soap and water, or designated solution per hospital SOP. Do not use powders or lotions, rinse well.
- (c)   Note color, character and odor of urine
  - (i)   Empty catheter bag every 8 hours or as directed by SOP/physician's order
  - (ii)   Ensure drainage spout does not contact contaminated surface.
  - (iii)   Measure and record I&O as ordered
  - (iv)   Observe patient for fever, chills or a sudden onset of pain
  - (v)   Apply topical antibiotic ointment to meatus, as ordered
  - (vi)   Check catheter frequently for patency and drainage of urine
  - (vii)   Secure catheter to patient to avoid pulling or pressure
  - (viii)   Clamp catheter temporarily if urine bag must be elevated higher then bladder. This prevents urine from draining back into bladder.
  - (ix)   Drainage system tubing should extend straight down from bed to drainage bag

NOTE: Any loops hanging down from bed level may promote stasis of urine, leading to infection.

TERMINAL LEARNING OBJECTIVE

Given a standard fully stocked M5 Bag or Combat Medic Vest System, oxygen, suction and ventilation equipment (if available). You encounter a casualty with symptoms of a skin disorder. No other injury (ies) or anaphylaxis symptoms are present, treat skin disorders IAW *Basic Trauma Life Support, Emergency Care in the Streets, Adult Health Nursing, Basic Nursing: A Critical Thinking Approach, Habif's Clinical Dermatology*

Assess for Skin Disorders

Temperature

Skin color

(1)	Lips
(2)	Oral membranes
(3)	Sclera
(4)	Conjunctiva
(5)	Palms and soles of feet

Skin integrity - palpate with gloved hands

(1)	Is the skin intact or not?
(2)	Texture (e.g., smoothness, and roughness)

Moist/dry

Skin lesion identification:

(1) **Primary lesions** are early skin changes that have not yet undergone natural evolution or change caused by manipulation. These are the best clues to diagnosis.

    (a) A macula is flat; color varies from white to brown to red to purple, and small (< 1 cm). A patch is a large macule (> 1 cm). Examples include freckles, flat moles, and tattoos.

    (b) A papule is a solid, elevated lesion usually < 1 cm. A plaque is a plateau-like lesion > 1 cm or a group of confluent papules. Examples include warts, some moles and some types of skin cancer

    (c) A nodule is a palpable, solid lesion >1-2 cm, elevated. Larger nodules (>2 cm) are called tumors. Examples include cysts or lipomas

    (d) A vesicle is a circumscribed, elevated lesion containing serous fluid that is < 1 cm; if > 1 cm, it is called a bulla (blister). Vesicles or bullae are commonly caused by primary irritants, allergic contact dermatitis, physical trauma, sunburn, insect bites

    (e) Pustules are superficial and elevated lesions containing pus < 1 cm. They may result from infection or seropurulent evolution of vesicles or bullae. Some causes are impetigo, acne and folliculitis

    (f) Wheals (hives) are transient, elevated lesions caused by localized edema. Wheals are a common allergic reaction, e.g., from drug eruptions, insect stings or bites, or sensitivity to cold, heat, pressure, or sunlight.

(g) Purpura is a general term referring to areas of extravasated blood. Petechiae are small-circumscribed punctate foci of extravasation, whereas ecchymoses (bruising) are larger confluent areas of extravasation. The term hematoma refers to an area of massive bleeding into the skin and underlying tissues

(8) Telangiectasias are dilated superficial blood vessels. They appear as red, threadlike lines. They may occur in certain systemic diseases or in long-term therapy with topical corticosteroids

(2) Secondary lesions result when primary lesions undergo a natural evolution

(a) Scales are particles of epithelium. Common scaling diseases are psoriasis and superficial fungal infections

(b) Crusts (scabs) consist of dried serum, blood, or pus. Crusting occurs in many inflammatory and infectious diseases

(c) Erosion is focal loss of part or all of the epidermis. It often occurs with herpes viral diseases

(d) Ulcers are focal loss of the epidermis and at least part of the dermis. When ulcers result from physical trauma or acute bacterial infection, the cause usually is apparent. Less obvious causes include chronic bacterial and fungal infections

(e) Excoriation is a linear or hollowed-out crusted area caused by scratching, rubbing, or picking

(f) Lichenification is a thickened skin area with accentuated skin markings

(g) Atrophy manifests as paper-thin, wrinkled skin. It occurs in the aged, after long-term use of topical potent corticosteroids, and sometimes after burns

(h) Scars are areas of fibrous tissue that replace normal skin after destruction of some of the dermis. Scars may be caused by burns or cuts or less commonly by systemic diseases

Presence of skin lesions

(1) Identify type of lesion
(2) Excretions
    (a) Color, odor, amount
    (b) Thick, oily etc.
(3) Size, does it change over time?
(4) Location

Turgor and mobility

(1) Turgor checks the hydration status of the patient

(2)   Pinch skin to form dent on back of patient's hand, abdomen, or sternum. Release skin and note how long it takes to return to normal position

Edema

(1)   Common sites are - face, eyelids, ankles, feet, sacral and scapular area

(2)   Indications of edema are - skin puffiness, tautness, or hardness

(3)   Types of edema - press in on area with thumb for 5 seconds and release

    (a)   Trace or shallow - slight indention that disappears (1+ second)

    (b)   Pitting - deep indentation that remains visible for several seconds (3-4 + seconds)

    (c)   Dependent - gravity causes fluid to pool in areas lowest to the earth.

Identify and Manage Viral Disorders of the Skin

Herpes simplex:

An infection from the herpes simplex virus (HSV) is characterized by one or many clusters of small vesicles filled with clear fluid on slightly raised inflammatory bases

(1)   Signs and symptoms

    (a)   The lesions may appear anywhere on the skin or mucosa but are most frequent around the mouth, on the lips, on the conjunctiva and in the genital area

    (b)   Incubation period is 2-20 days. Asymptomatic „carriers" shed the virus and spread the disease

    (c)   After a prodromal period; tingling, discomfort or itching and small tense vesicles appear on an erythematous base

    (d)   Single clusters vary in size from 0.5 to 1.5 cm, but groups may coalesce

    (e)   The vesicles persist for a few days, and then begin to dry, forming a thin yellowish crust or ulcer

    (f)   Primary (initial) infection is generally the most severe, with fever, lymphadenopathy and urinary symptoms (if the outbreak is genital)

    (g)   A herpetic whitlow is a HSV infection of the fingers, resulting from an inoculation of HSV through a cutaneous break. Common in health care workers. Symptoms include swelling and pain over lesions around the finger nail.

(2)   Treatment

    (a)   Healing generally occurs in 8 to 12 days after onset

    (b)   Individual herpetic lesions usually heal completely, but recurrent lesions at the same site may cause atrophy and scarring

(c)   Antiviral medications (acyclovir) are used for initial outbreaks, recurrent infections and suppressive therapy

(d)   Secondary bacterial infections are treated with systemic antibiotics

(e)   Avoid sexual intercourse while genital lesions are present. Viral shedding may occur even if patient is symptom free. Discuss condom usage with all genital herpes patients

(f)   Refer the patient to a MD/PA for treatment

Herpes zoster

(Shingles) An infection with varicella-zoster virus primarily involving the dorsal root ganglia and characterized by vesicular eruption and neuralgic pain in the dermatome of the affected root ganglia

(1)   Signs and symptoms
- (a)   Pain along the site of the future eruption usually precedes the rash by 2 to 3 days
- (b)   Characteristic crops of vesicles on an erythematous base then appear, following the cutaneous distribution of one dermatome
- (c)   The involved zone is usually hyperesthetic, and pain may be severe
- (d)   Eruptions occur most often in the thoracic or lumbar region and are unilateral
- (e)   Lesions usually continue to form for about 3 to 5 days
- (f)   Crusting occurs by 7-10 days and resolves by 14-21 days

(2)   Treatment
- (a)   Locally applied wet compresses are soothing, but systemic analgesics are often necessary
- (b)   Oral antiviral medications are used for treatment of herpes zoster
- (c)   Refer the patient to a MD/PA for treatment

Identify and Manage Bacterial Disorders

Cellulitis-

An acute infection of the skin and subcutaneous tissues. It may arise from an entry of bacteria through the skin (i.e. laceration, puncture wound) or extension from an abscess. Cellulitis is a serious disease because of the possibility of the infection spreading to the lymphatic and blood systems resulting in bacteremia and sepsis.

(1)   Signs and Symptoms
- (a)   Infection is most common in the lower extremities
- (b)   The major findings are local erythema and tenderness, frequently with lymphangitis and regional lymphadenopathy
- (c)   The skin is hot, red, and edematous

(d)   Vesicles and bullae may develop and rupture, occasionally with necrosis of the involved skin

(e)   Systemic manifestations (fever, chills, tachycardia) may precede the cutaneous findings by several hours, but many patients do not appear ill

(f)   Local abscesses form occasionally, requiring incision and drainage

(2)   Treatment

(a)   Oral antibiotic therapy to cover streptococci and staphylococci is required as first line outpatient therapy. Keflex 500 mg four times a day or Dynapen 500 mg four times a day. For penicillin allergic patients; Erythromycin 500mg four times a day is generally used. Duration of therapy is 10-14 days.

(b)   For severe infections, which require hospitalization, Ancef 2 grams intravenously four times a day is used. For penicillin allergic patients, clindamycin 150-300 mg intravenously is given

(c)   Immobilization and elevation of the affected area help reduce edema, and cool, wet dressings relieve local discomfort

(d)   Refer patient to MD/PA for treatment

Impetigo: Impetigo is a superficial skin infection

(1)   Signs and Symptoms: Impetigo may occur on normal skin, especially on the legs in children. Impetigo usually occurs near the lips or nasolabial folds

(a)   Lesions initially are pea-sized papules, becoming vesicular and rupturing, leaving the classic „honey-colored crusts"

(b)   Regional lymphadenopathy is seen in the majority of cases

(c)   Constitutional symptoms are absent

(2)   Treatment

(a)   Application of mupirocin ointment 3 times daily has been effective in treating impetigo

(b)   Patients showing no response to mupirocin in 3 to 5 days should be treated systemically. Because most cases are caused by either streptococci or staph- erythromycin is the drug of choice. Adults are given 250 mg four times a day

(c)   Impetigo is extremely contagious. Avoidance of patients' towels or linens is crucial to avoid the spread of infection

(d)   Refer patient to MD/PA for treatment

Cutaneous Abscesses:

(1)   Signs and symptoms include localized collections of pus causing fluctuant soft tissue swelling surrounded by erythema.

(2)   Treatment

(a)   Incision of the fluctuant area, thorough draining of pus with meticulous probing
(b)   Pack the cavity loosely with a gauze wick that is removed 24 to 48 h later
(c)   Local heat and elevation may resolve tissue inflammation
(d)   Refer patient to MD/PA for incision and drainage

Folliculitis:

Superficial or deep bacterial infection and inflammation of the hair follicles
(1)   Signs and symptoms
(a)   A superficial pustule or inflammatory nodule surrounding a hair follicle
(b)   The condition may follow or accompany other skin infections
(c)   Chronic low-grade irritation or inflammation without significant infection may occur when stiff hairs in the bearded area emerge from the follicle, curve, and reenter the skin (pseudofolliculitis barbae)
(2)   Treatment
(a)   Topical antibiotics and antiseptics (e.g., chlorhexidine) may be useful adjuncts to systemic therapy but should not be used without concomitant systemic treatment
(b)   Treatment with systemic antibiotics may be indicated
(c)   Refer patient to MD/PA for treatment

Furuncle (Boil)

Acute, tender, perifollicular inflammatory nodules resulting from infection by staphylococci. The condition often occurs in healthy young persons.
(1)   Signs and symptoms
(a)   Furuncles occur most frequently on the neck, breasts, face, and buttocks but are most painful when on skin closely attached to underlying structures (e.g., on the nose, ear, or fingers)
(b)   The initial nodule becomes a .5-2 cm pustule that discharges a core of necrotic tissue and pus
(2)   Treatment
(a)   Incision and drainage or application of liquid soap containing either chlorhexidine gluconate with isopropyl alcohol or 2 to 3% chloroxylenol, which may be prophylactic but is not therapeutic
(b)   A single furuncle is treated with intermittent hot compresses to allow the lesion to point and either drain spontaneously or incised and drained
(c)   Facial furuncles should be managed closely, due to the possibility of retrograde spread of infection through cranial channels
(d)   Patients with furuncles are usually treated with systemic antibiotics. Usually a penicillinase-resistant penicillin is

required, such as cloxacillin 250 to 500 mg P.O. qid, or a cephalosporin, such as cephalexin in the same dosage
(e)   Refer patient to MD/PA for treatment

Carbuncle

A cluster of furuncles with subcutaneous spread of staphylococcal infection, resulting in deep suppuration, often extensive local sloughing, slow healing, and a large scar
(1)   Signs and symptoms
    (a)   Carbuncles occur most frequently in males and most commonly on the nape of the neck
    (b)   Carbuncles develop more slowly than single furuncles and may be accompanied by fever and prostration
(2)   Treatment is the same as for clusters of furuncles (see above)
(3)   Refer patient to MD/PA for treatment

Bites

1-3 million animal bites to humans occur annually in the U.S. Dog bites represent 70-90% of all bites. Cat bites represent 7-20% and have a higher incidence of infection. Human and rodent bites make up the remainder of bites.
(1)   Signs and symptoms
    (a)   The extremities are involved in 75% of cases when victims handle or attempt to avoid the animal. Head and neck injuries are the next most common
    (b)   Wounds should be described as to size, location and type. Include diagrams. If infected, describe adenopathy and diagram extent of cellulitis
    (c)   These organisms are resistant to many antibiotics but are generally sensitive to ampicillin and penicillin
    (d)   All bite injuries are potentially dangerous and can cause significant infection
(2)   Treatment
    (a)   Wash with warm soapy water
    (b)   Provide aggressive and meticulous wound care
    (c)   Provide tetanus prophylaxis, as indicated
    (d)   Systemic antibiotics for anaerobic and aerobic organisms are given. The type of antibiotic given is dependent on type of animal involved
    (e)   Review rabies postexposure prophylaxis guidelines. Exposure is defined as an open bite or wound in contact with body fluids
    (f)   Review for possibility of hepatitis B or C transmission in human bites and provide immunoprophylaxis if necessary
    (g)   Refer all bite wounds to a MD/PA for assessment and treatment

Felon

Infection of the distal fat pad of a digit. The most common site is the distal pulp, which may be involved centrally, laterally, and apically. Staph aureus is the usual bacteria involved

(1)   Signs and symptoms
    (a)   The area between pulp spaces ordinarily limit the spread of infection, resulting in an abscess, which creates pressure of adjacent tissues
    (b)   The underlying bone, joint, or flexor tendons may become infected, and intense throbbing pain and a swollen pulp are present
(2)   Treatment
    (a)   Treatment involves prompt incision and drainage
    (b)   Systemic antibiotics are generally given
    (c)   Wound should be checked in 1-3 days
    (d)   Refer patient to MD/PA for treatment

Identify and Manage Inflammatory Disorders

Contact Dermatitis

Contact dermatitis can be subdivided into allergic contact dermatitis and irritant contact dermatitis
(1)   Primary irritants may damage normal skin or irritate existing dermatitis
(2)   Allergic contact dermatitis patients may become allergic to substances that they have sometimes used for years or to drugs used to treat skin diseases
(3)   Examples of agents that may cause contact dermatitis
    (a)   Medications- topical
    (b)   Plants-poison oak, poison ivy
    (c)   Chemicals used in the manufacture of shoes and clothing, metal compounds, dyes, and cosmetics
    (d)   Industrial agents
    (e)   Sensitivity to rubber and latex in gloves is a particular problem for many health professionals
    (f)   Sensitivity to latex condoms may preclude their use in some men
    (g)   Photodermatitis occurs after sunlight exposure of a patient wearing photosensitizers that exaggerates the suns effect. Aftershave lotions, sunscreens, and topical sulfonamides are commonly responsible for photoallergic contact dermatitis
    (h)   Perfumes
(4)   Signs and Symptoms
    (a)   Transient redness to severe swelling with bullae
    (b)   Pruritus and vesiculation are common

        (c)   Any skin surface exposed to an irritant or sensitizing substance

        (d)   Typically, the dermatitis is limited to the site of contact but may later spread

        (e)   Vesicles and bullae may rupture, ooze, and crust

        (f)   As inflammation subsides, scaling and some temporary thickening of the skin occur

        (g)   Continued exposure to the causative agent (e.g., irritation from or allergy to a topical drug, excoriation, and infection) may perpetuate the dermatitis

(5)   Diagnosis

        (a)   Typical skin changes and a history of exposure facilitate diagnosis

        (b)   The patient's occupation, hobbies, household duties, vacations, clothing, topical drug use, cosmetics, and spouse's activities must be considered

        (c)   Knowing the characteristics of irritants or topical allergens and the typical distribution of lesions is helpful

        (d)   The site of the initial lesion is often an important clue

(6)   Treatment: Unless the causative agent is identified and removed, treatment will be ineffective. Patients with photodermatitis should also avoid the photosensitizing chemical or exposure to light

        (a)   In acute dermatitis, gauze or thin cloths dipped in water and applied to the lesions (30 min 4 to 6 times/day) are soothing and cooling

        (b)   An oral corticosteroid (e.g., predispose 60 mg/day) may be given (if not contraindicated) for 7 to 14 days in extensive cases, or even in limited cases when facial inflammation is present. The prednisone dose can be decreased by 10 to 20 mg q 3 to 4 days

        (c)   Topical corticosteroids are not helpful in the blistering phase, but once the dermatitis is less acute, a topical corticosteroid cream or ointment can be rubbed in gently three times daily

        (d)   Antihistamines are ineffective in suppressing allergic contact dermatitis but help the itch

Pruritus (Itching)

A sensation that the patient instinctively attempts to relieve by scratching or rubbing

(1)   Etiology: Pruritus is a symptom and not a disease. It may accompany a primary skin disease or a systemic disease. Skin diseases causing severe pruritus and lesions include scabies, pediculosis, insect bites, urticaria, atopic dermatitis, and contact dermatitis

(2)   Systemic conditions that cause generalized pruritus, usually without skin lesions, include

    (a)   Liver disease

    (b)   Kidney disease

    (c)   Uremia-excessive amounts of urea and other waste products in the blood

    (d)   Pregnancy

    (e)   Medications

(3)   Signs and symptoms:

    (a)   Persistent scratching may produce redness, linear urticarial papules, and excoriation of preexisting papules, fissures, and elongated crusts along scratch lines, which may obscure the underlying disease

    (b)   Lichenification and pigmentation may also result from prolonged scratching and rubbing. Occasionally, patients who complain of severe generalized pruritus have few signs of scratching or rubbing the skin

(4)   Treatment: The cause of generalized pruritus should be sought and corrected. If no skin disease is apparent, a systemic disorder or drug-related cause should be sought

    (a)   If feasible, all drugs should be stopped

    (b)   Clothing that is irritating (e.g., woolens) or tight should be avoided

    (c)   Bathing should be brief, as it may aggravate generalized pruritus, especially if the patient has dry skin; lukewarm (not hot) water should be used

    (d)   Emollients (e.g., white petrolatum or other oil-based products) are good moisturizers to apply after bathing while the skin is still wet (excess water should be blotted)

    (e)   Topical corticosteroids seldom alleviate generalized pruritus (without dermatitis) but may be useful if used with lubricants in elderly patients with dry skin

    (f)   If a drug has been ruled out as the cause of pruritus, hydroxyzine (10 to 50 mg P.O. q 4 h prn) may be prescribed. If antihistamines are helpful, their sedative effect may be the reason

Bulla (blister)

    (1)   Definition - a large blister or skin vesicle filled with fluid below the epidermis

    (2)   Causes

           (a)   Thermal or chemical burns (2nd degree)

           (b)   Friction or pressure (e.g., poorly fitted shoes, rug burn)

           (c)   Ruptured blood vessels due to trauma

           (d)   Herpes simplex (fever blister)

    (3)   Signs and symptoms

           (a)   Large elevated fluid filled lesion greater than 1 cm in diameter

           (b)   Discoloration at borders of blister, may be red or pale pink

           (c)   Pain and tenderness with palpation or pressure. Mostly occurs on feet

    (4)   Treatment

           (a)   Avoid aggravating area by removing cause as soon as possible (e.g., tight shoes/boots, wet socks)

           (b)   "DO NOT" lance blister unless unable to remove cause (e.g., blister located on foot during a road march)

           (c)   If cause can not be removed, lance bottom of blister with a sterile needle or scalpel, and allow to drain

           (d)   Keep area covered and clean. Build up dressing around blister to prevent friction

Identify and Manage Fungal Infections of the Skin

Fungal infections are common on the feet and the body

    (1)   Fungal infections may be pruritic or asymptomatic. Occasionally there is tenderness and inflammation

    (2)   Symptoms- depend on the location

           (a)   Scalp (tinea capitus)- alopecia, scaling, swelling and occasional purulent discharge

           (b)   Feet (tinea pedis)- scaling, thickened soles, occasional blisters

           (c)   Skin (tinea corporis)- inflammation and scaling

    (3)   Skin (Tinea Corporis)

           (a)   Erythematous plaque with central clearing and sharp margins

           (b)   The organism may persist indefinitely, causing intermittent remissions and exacerbations of a gradually extending lesion with a scaling, slightly raised border

           (c)   Intense inflammation with or without pustules may be present

           (d)   Treatment- Most skin infections respond very well to topical antifungal preparations, such micatin, tinactin or lamisil. Resistant cases or those with widespread involvement require systemic antifungal therapy.

    (4)   Tinea pedis (Athlete's Foot)

    (a) Infections typically begin in the 3rd and 4th interdigital spaces and later involve the plantar surface of the arch

    (b) Toe web lesions often are macerated and have scaling borders; they may be vesicular

    (c) Acute flare-ups, with many vesicles and bullae, are common during warm   weather

    (d) Tinea pedis may be complicated by secondary bacterial infection, cellulitis, or lymphangitis, which may recur

    (e) Treatment- Interdigital infections can be successfully treated with topical agents. Good foot hygiene is essential. Interdigital spaces must be dried after bathing, macerated skin gently debrided, and a bland, drying antifungal powder (eg, miconazole) applied

    (f) Cure with topical treatment is difficult, but control may be obtained with long-term therapy. Recurrence is common after therapy is discontinued

  (5) Tinea capitis (Scalp): Tinea capitis mainly affects children. It is contagious and may become epidemic

    (a) Inflammation that is low-grade and persistent. Alopecia may occur with characteristic black dots on the scalp result from broken hairs

    (b) Treatment- topical treatment is not advised. Oral antifungal therapy is indicated

  (6) Tinea cruris (Jock Itch)

    (a) Typically, a ringed lesion extends from the crural fold over the adjacent upper inner thigh. Both sides may be affected

    (b) Scratch dermatitis and lichenification often occur. Lesions may be complicated by maceration, miliaria, secondary bacterial or candidal infection, and reactions to treatment

    (c) Recurrence is common because fungi may repeatedly infect susceptible persons. Flare-ups occur more often during summer, due to heat and humidity of the skin area

    (d) Tight clothing or obesity tends to favor growth of the organisms

    (e) Treatment- Topical therapy with a cream or lotion, as in tinea corporis, is often effective. Instruct the patient to keep the area as clean and dry as possible,

Identify and Manage Other Skin Disorders

Scabies

The arthropod itch mite causes the dermatitis scabies in humans. Transmission occurs between people via skin-to-skin contact or through bed linens and clothing

  (1) Signs and Symptoms

    (a) Intense itching, especially at night, with vesicles, papules and linear burrows which contain the mites and eggs

    (b) Lesions prominent around finger webs, elbows, buttocks and genital area

    (c)   Complications are generally due to infection of lesions that are broken from scratching

(2)   Treatment

    (a)   Treatment should include the patient, sexual partners, household members and caregivers

    (b)   Overnight applications of topical medications have proven to be the most effective

    (c)   Bag patient's linen separately. Instruct the patient to wash bedding in HOT water

Lice

(1)   Three types:

    (a)   Pediculosis Pubis

        (i)   Infestation in the pubic region

        (ii)   Spread by intimate contact, often sexual

        (iii)   The lice survive for about one day off the host.

    (b)   Pediculosis capitis

        (i)   Infestation on the scalp

        (ii)   Spread by casual contact and by fomites such as shared combs or hats

        (iii)   Survive only a few days off the host.

    (c)   Pediculosis corporis

        (i)   Usually found on clothing, particularly in the seams around warm areas

        (ii)   Come onto the skin only to feed

(2)   Signs and Symptoms

    (a)   Pediculosis Pubis

        (i)   Complains of perineal pruritus

        (ii)   Examination shows adult lice attached to the skin and nits attached to hair shafts

        (iii)   Blue macules around the thighs and pubic area may occur at sites where the organism is feeding

    (b)   Pediculosis capitis

        (i)   Complains of itching of the scalp or eyelashes

        (ii)   Examination shows adult lice in hair

        (iii)   Nits at the base of the hair shaft, macules, wheals, and excoriations are present

    (c)   Pediculosis corporis

        (i)   Complains of diffuse pruritus (especially if there is evidence of generally poor hygiene)

        (ii)   Examination reveals erythematous macules, wheals, and excoriations, often with superinfection

        (iii)   Lice are found in clothing rather than on body

(3)   Treatment of Pediculosis pubis, capitis, corporis

    (a)   Overnight applications of topical medications have proven to be the most effective

    (b)   Bag patient's linen separately. Instruct the patient to wash bedding in HOT water

(c)   Hats, combs, and brushes should be thoroughly cleaned before being reused

(d)   Sexual contacts of patients should be also be treated and close contact of patient with pediculosis capitis and corporis should be examined for lice.

(e)   Since both scabies and pediculosis may be sexually transmitted, examination for other sexually transmitted diseases should be performed and a serologic test for syphilis (VDRL or other) obtain

TERMINAL LEARNING OBJECTIVE

Given a standard fully stocked M5 Bag or Combat Medic Vest System, oxygen, suction and ventilation equipment (if available), selected medications, and documentation forms. You encounter a casualty complaining of infectious disease and/or immunological symptoms. No other injury(ies) are present.

Review Concepts Associated with Infectious Diseases

Public health principles relative to infectious diseases

   (1)   All humans are susceptible to infectious disease
   (2)   Individuals display varying susceptibilities to infection
   (3)   When dealing with infectious diseases, the soldier medic must consider the needs of the casualty, potential consequence on public health and his own health protection
   (4)   The soldier medic should think of the consequences of the patients' contact with family members, roommates and friends

Infectious agents

   (1)   Bacteria- unicellular microorganisms
   (2)   Viruses- submicroscopic organism. Able to replicate only in a living cell
   (3)   Fungi- spore bearing plants
   (4)   Rickettsia- microorganisms, which combine qualities of bacteria and viruses
   (5)   Helminths (worms)- various invertebrates, having round or flattened bodies

Terminology of the immune system

   (1)   Antibodies- a protein produced by lymphocytes in response to infectious agents
   (2)   Antigen- A substance which causes the formation of an antibody
   (3)   Epitope- a specific site where an antibody binds. May be numerous epitopes on one antigen
   (4)   Leukocytes- White blood cells
       (a)   Five types:
          (i)   Lymphocytes
             * T cells - Divide rapidly when exposed to antigen. May assist in destroying foreign protein
             * B cells - circulate in immature form, activated when exposed to antigen
          (ii) Monocytes
             * Ingest dead or damaged cells via phagocytosis (absorption of foreign bodies in the bloodstream)
             * Provide immunological defenses against infectious organisms
          (iii) Neutrophils

                        *   Essential for phagocytosis

(iv)   Basophils
- *   Increased number during healing phase and inflammation
- *   Immediate immune response to external antigens

(v)   Eosinophils
- *   Increase numbers in certain diseases, especially infections by helminths and allergies

Host defense mechanisms

(1)   Nonspecific immune system defenses
- (a)   Skin
  - (i)   Effectively bars invading microorganisms
  - (ii)   Some exceptions occur, as with human papillomavirus (causative agent of warts) which can invade normal skin
  - (iii)   Normal dermal flora - alteration of this flora can lead to overgrowth of inherently pathogenic microorganisms
- (b)   Respiratory system
  - (i)   Inhaled microorganisms must penetrate the filter system of the upper airways and tracheobroncial tree
  - (ii)   Coughing also helps remove organisms
  - (iii)   Smoking greatly impairs effectiveness
  - (iv)   These defense mechanisms can be overcome by large numbers of organisms or by compromised effectiveness resulting from air pollutants
- (c)   Inflammatory response
  - (i)   Directs immune system components to injury or infection sites and is manifested by increased blood supply and vascular permeability
  - (ii)   Microorganisms are engulfed by phagocytic cells in an attempt to contain the infection

(2)   Specific immune system defenses
- (a)   Humoral immunity
  - (i)   Component of the immune system involving antibodies
  - (ii)   Recognizes antigens associated with microorganisms or foreign substances
  - (iii)   Recognition is coupled with ability to initiate appropriate actions against these microorganisms or foreign substances
- (b)   Cell-mediated immunity
  - (i)   Phagocytic and/or cytotoxic cells play major role
  - (ii)   Antibody plays minor role

	(iii)	Macrophages and neutrophils important in combating bacteria
	(iv)	T cells essential to elimination of virus-infected cells

General Assessment of Suspected Infectious or Communicable Disease

Primary assessment

(1)   Ensure open airway
(2)   Assess breathing
(3)   Assess circulation

Secondary assessment (specific to infectious disease)

(1)   History of present illness
(2)   Past medical history
       (a)   Chronic infections, inflammation
       (b)   Medications
       (c)   Medical and surgical history
(3)   Detailed history and physical
       (a)   Vital signs
       (b)   Assess skin
             (i)   Temperature
             (ii)   Turgor (hydration)
             (iii)   Color (jaundice)
             (iv)   Abnormal lesions
       (c)   Assess Head, Ears, Eyes, Neck, and Throat (HEENT)
       (d)   Assess neck
             (i)   Lymphadenopathy - localized or generalized enlargement of lymph nodes or lymph vessels
             (ii)   Rigidity
       (e)   Assess for abnormal breath sounds
       (f)   Assess abdomen
             (i)   Tenderness
             (ii)   Rebound
             (iii)   Guarding or organomegaly
       (g)   Assess extremities for edema, pain and joint range of motion (ROM)

Assess and Treat Eye, Ear, Nose, Throat, and Respiratory Complaints

Conjunctivitis (pink eye)

(1)   Infection of the membrane lining the eyelids (conjunctiva)
(2)   Signs and Symptoms- may be unilateral or bilateral
       (a)   Pruritus
       (b)   Burning
       (c)   Itching
       (d)   Swelling
       (e)   Excessive purulent discharge or tearing
       (f)   Redness

(3)   Provide medical care
- (a)   Perform visual acuity before any treatment is initiated
- (b)   Ensure eye is not injured and no foreign body is present
- (c)   Administer ophthalmic ointments or solutions for conjunctivitis as ordered by MD/PA
- (d)   Use universal precautions gloves), conjunctivitis is very contagious

Pharyngitis (sore throat)

(1)   The majority of sore throat complaints are viral in origin, not bacterial

(2)   Most common bacteria causing pharyngitis is group A Beta hemolytic streptococcus

(3)   Signs and symptoms
- (a)   Often difficult to clinically differentiate between viral and bacterial infections
- (b)   Patients with a bacterial (strep) infection may present with:
  - (i)   Sudden on set of sore throat
  - (ii)   Painful swallowing
  - (iii)   Chills and fever
  - (iv)   Headache, nausea, vomiting and abdominal pain are common associated symptoms
- (c)   Physical examination of patients with strep throat reveals
  - (i)   Foul smelling breath
  - (ii)   Beefy red throat
  - (iii)   Tonsillar exudate
  - (iv)   Enlarged, tender anterior cervical lymph nodes. There is no posterior cervical adenopathy.
  - (v)   Patient may have petechiae on the palate and strawberry tongue
- (d)   Patient with a viral pharyngitis usually present with a more vesicular and petechial pattern on the soft palate and tonsils and no exudate
- (e)   Throat culture remains the most effective method for diagnosis

(4)   Provide medical care
- (a)   Symptomatic treatment
  - (i)   Gargling with warm salt water
  - (ii)   Drinking warm liquids
  - (iii)   Rest
  - (iv)   Consider IV hydration in patients who are unable to tolerate oral fluids or who become dehydrated
- (b)   Antibiotics
  - (i)   Drug of choice for strep throat is penicillin. Ampicillin or amoxicillin may also be used.
  - (ii)   May also consider cephalosporin
  - (iii)   Erythromycin is drug of choice for patients allergic to penicillin
  - (iv)   Oral medications usually administered for 10 days even though pain from sore throat may resolve in 24-48 hours

(v)   Refer to MD/PA for appropriate therapy

(c)   Untreated strep throat (group A B – hemolytic streptococcus) is associated with significant sequela in the form of acute rheumatic fever or acute glomerulonephritis. Because of this, early diagnosis and treatment of strep throat is essential.

(d)   Prevent spread
(i)   Handwash
(ii)   Avoid using same utensils or drinking from same container
(iii)   Avoid close contact

(e)   Infectious mononucleosis
(i)   Acute viral infection is primarily caused by an Epstein-Barr virus (EBV). Infrequent causes are Cytomegalovirus (CMV) and Human Immunodeficiency Virus (HIV)
(ii)   Humans are the sole source, with transmission by close contact. Incubation period is 3-7 weeks.
(iii)   Assessment findings
*   High fever
*   Swollen lymph glands
*   Sore throat
*   Fatigue
*   Persistent headache
*   Acute phase lasts 1-3 weeks, with complete recovery expected in 6-8 weeks
*   Most serious complication is splenic rupture due to an enlarged spleen, combined with physical activity. Limited activity during the acute phase is required. All soldiers must be assessed by an MD/PA for suspected mono cases.
(iv)   Provide care
*   Uncomplicated acute infectious mononucleosis usually only requires supportive therapy
*   Consider Tylenol for fever and pain
*   Warm salt water gargles for sore throat
*   Patient should get ample bed rest. Isolation is unnecessary because EBV shedding continues after the acute illness
*   Recovery occurs in a few weeks; however, some people take months to regain former level of energy

Influenza

    (1)   Viral infection of the respiratory tract

    (2)   Flu vaccine is available annually. Influenza is self-limited in healthy individuals, but its potentially severe consequences must be stressed to elderly or chronically ill patients to ensure their annual vaccination.

    (3)   Assessment findings

        (a)   Fever- may be high (up to 103 degrees)- rapid onset and may last 3-5 days

        (b)   Cough- usually nonproductive. If a secondary bacterial infection occurs, cough turns productive with purulent sputum

        (c)   Headache

        (d)   Muscle aches- may to tender to palpation

        (e)   Shortness of breath

        (f)   Chills

        (g)   Sweating

        (h)   Fatigue

        (i)   Nausea and vomiting

        (j)   Joint stiffness and aches

        (k)   Nausea, vomiting

    (4)   Provide medical care

        (a)   Because influenza is a viral infection, antibiotics are not helpful

        (b)   Bed rest

        (c)   Provide analgesics for muscles aches

        (d)   Provide oral or intravenous fluids

        (e)   Symptoms may last 7 - 10 days

        (f)   Notify MD/PA if:

            (i)   Symptoms increase

            (ii)   Fever is present

            (iii)   Unable to keep food or fluids down

Cough

    (1)   Sudden, forceful release of air from the lungs

        (a)   Helps clear material

        (b)   May produce and expel mucus and/or pus - productive cough

        (c)   Minor irritations in throat can start cough reflex though normal mucus is only material expelled - dry cough

    (2)   Common causes include:

        (a)   Smoking

        (b)   Common cold or flu

        (c)   Allergies

        (d)   Bacterial infection

        (e)   Viral infection

        (f)   Asthma

        (g)   Emphysema

    (3)   Assessment Findings

        (a)   Shortness of breath requires immediate evaluation.

        (b)   Productive or nonproductive cough - Productive may be rusty/blood-streaked, yellow-green or yellow sputum
        (c)   Elevated temperature
        (d)   Chest may be clear to auscultation or have abnormal breath sounds (wheezing, rhonchi or crackles)

(4)   Provide medical care
        (a)   Increase air humidity, if available
        (b)   Inform patient to drink extra fluids
        (c)   Consider an expectorant to help liquefy secretions
        (d)   Consider a decongestant if cough is accompanied by runny nose
        (e)   Consider antihistamines if caused by allergy or sinus infection
        (f)   Dry tickling coughs can be relieved by lozenges

(5)   Notify MD/PA if:
        (a)   Violent cough begins suddenly or high-pitched sound (stridor)
        (b)   Produce blood
        (c)   Shortness of breath and/or difficulty breathing
        (d)   Abnormal breath sounds are heard on auscultation
        (e)   Fever or abdominal swelling
        (f)   Unintentional weight loss
        (g)   Thick, foul-smelling, rusty, or greenish mucous
        (h)   Lasts more than 10 days

Pneumonia
(1)   Inflammation of lungs caused by an infection
(2)   Prevention
        (a)   Vaccination (flu, pneumovax) may be helpful in preventing some types of pneumonia
        (b)   Coughing and deep breathing

Bronchitis

(1)   Inflammation of the bronchi
(2)   Prevention
        (a)   Early recognition
        (b)   Treat small airway disease
        (c)   Smoking cessation

Viral Upper Respiratory Infection (Common Cold)

(1)   Contagious viral infection of the upper respiratory tract. Transmission may occur through air droplets (sneezing) or lack of handwashing
(2)   Assessment Findings (usually minimal)
        (a)   Runny nose
        (b)   Nasal congestion
        (c)   Sneezing
        (d)   Sore throat
        (e)   Cough
        (f)   Muscle aches
        (g)   Headache

    (h) Low grade fever (100 F or lower)
  (3) Provide medical care
    (a) Consider antihistamine and/or decongestant for nasal congestion
    (b) Consider Tylenol for minor aches and pains
    (c) Patient should get able bed rest
    (d) Instruct patient to drink plenty of fluids
    (e) Patient should return to MTF if:
      (i) Develop temperature greater than 101F
      (ii) Develop a productive cough
      (iii) Symptoms do not begin to improve within the next 2-3 days

Assess and Treat Gastrointestinal (GI) Complaints

Nausea/Vomiting

  (1) Nausea is the sensation leading to the urge to vomit
  (2) Vomit is to force the contents of the stomach up through the esophagus and out of the mouth
  (3) A common cause is a viral infection. Assessment findings include:
    (a) Presence of absence of abdominal pain
    (b) Description of emesis
    (c) Fever
  (4) Provide care
    (a) Instruct patient to drink clear fluids for 24 hours. Solids should be increased as tolerated.
    (b) Patient should get bed rest
    (c) Instruct patient to return to MTF if:
      (i) Blood is in vomitus
      (ii) Increasing abdominal pain
      (iii) Nausea/vomiting persists for greater than 24 hours

Diarrhea

  (1) Frequent passage of unformed, watery stool
  (2) Infectious diarrheal disease can be grouped:
    (a) Viruses
    (b) Bacteria
    (c) Parasites
    (d) Funguses
  (3) Assessment findings include:
    (a) Abdominal cramps
    (b) Fever
  (4) Provide care
    (a) Observe good hygiene. Wash hands frequently.
    (b) Consider Imodium (only if non bloody) or Pepto-Bismol
      (i) May be given to the patient for the symptomatic control of diarrhea
      (ii) Best treatment is NOT to interfere with the mechanical cleansing of the GI tract

(c)   If diarrhea is not controlled in 24-48 hours with normal medications, refer patient to MD/PA for assessment

Gastroenteritis

(1)   Inflammation of stomach and intestines due to bacterial or viral infection

(2)   Modes of transmission
    (a)   Fecal-oral
    (b)   Ingestion of infected food or non-potable water

(3)   Susceptibility and resistance
    (a)   Travelers into endemic areas are more susceptible
    (b)   Populations in disaster areas, where water supplies are contaminated, are susceptible
    (c)   Native populations in endemic areas are generally resistant

(4)   Assessment findings include:
    (a)   Nausea/Vomiting
    (b)   Diarrhea
    (c)   Fever
    (d)   Abdominal pain and cramping
    (e)   Diarrhea
    (f)   Heartburn

(5)   Provide care
    (a)   Antibiotic therapy is usually not indicated
    (b)   Consider antidiarrheal medications, though not generally given because they may prolong infectious process
    (c)   Clear liquid diet

Assess and Treat a Fever, Headache, and Sinus Symptoms

Fever-

Fever is a common presenting symptom, accounting from 2-6 percent of adults presenting to hospital emergency rooms and clinics.

(1)   Fever can be due to:
    (a)   Infection: all causes, whether bacterial, viral or parasitic
    (b)   Trauma
    (c)   Immunologic: serum sickness or acute inflammatory arthritis
    (d)   Drug induced
    (e)   Vascular disorders: acute myocardial infarction, pulmonary emboli

(2)   Acute bacterial infection requires a timely diagnosis and treatment. The initial approach to evaluating a patient with an acute fever is detecting a treatable infection or excluding a bacterial infection with reasonable certainty.

(3)   Fever above 100 F must be evaluated by an MD/PA

(4)   Provide care
    (a)   Administer Tylenol or Motrin. The use of aspirin should not be used due to bleeding problems

      (b)   If fever is uncontrolled, seek methods of cooling patient. Such as cooling mats, tepid baths or showers.

Headache

(1)   Meningitis- an infection of the meninges (the membranes surrounding the brain)

      (a)   Causes:
- (i)   Bacterial
- (ii)   Viral
- (iii)   Fungal

      (c)   Signs and Symptoms
- (i)   Headache, sudden onset, severe, usually occipital
- (ii)   Fever
- (iii)   Chills
- (iv)   Photophobia
- (v)   Neck stiffness or nuchal rigidity (more pronounced on flexion)
- (vi)   Petechial rash - Bacterial
- (vii)   Altered mental status
- (viii)   Nausea and vomiting

      (d)   Provide medical care
- (i)   Protective measures should include BSI with surgical masks applied to casualties displaying suggestive signs/ symptoms
- (ii)   **Meningitis is a medical emergency. Delay in treatment will result in death.** Notify MD/PA immediately and evacuate
- (iii)   Initiate IV
- (iv)   Perform serial neurological examinations

Sinusitis

(1)   Disorder involving infection and/or inflammation of one or more of the paranasal sinuses. The maxillary sinuses are the most frequently affected. Factors predisposing to sinusitis are upper respiratory infection, smoking, allergies and nasal polyps.

(2)   Assessment findings include:
- (a)   Headache
- (b)   Purulent nasal discharge
- (c)   Cough
- (d)   Pain in the sinus area with palpation or percussion
- (e)   Facial pain
- (f)   Pain may also be referred to the teeth. Patients may complain of a "toothache".

(3)   Provide medical care
- (a)   Administer analgesics to relieve pain
- (b)   Administer saline or decongestant nasal sprays to increase drainage
- (c)   Consider an expectorant/mucolytic to thin secretions and promote drainage

(d)   Antibiotic therapy is indicated for 10-21 days. Antibiotic
        choice is based on duration of symptoms and the
        individual patient
(e)   Refer patient to MD/PA for suspected sinus infections

Assess and Treat Hepatitis

Viral Hepatitis-

Management of viral hepatitis has been through major changes, therefore
knowledge of the various types is important. At least 7 major viruses have
been identified and cause the majority of disease
(1)   **Hepatitis A**- inflammation of liver caused by hepatitis A virus
        (a)   Seen worldwide and is a food and water-borne disease
        (b)   Spread by fecal-oral contact
(2)   Signs and symptoms
        (a)   Symptoms are similar to flu
                (i)   Fever
                (ii)   Weakness
        (b)   Jaundice of skin and eyes - liver is not able to filter bilirubin
                from blood
        (c)   Darkening of urine
        (d)   Clay colored stools
        (e)   Nausea and vomiting
(3)   Provide care
        (a)   Treatment is primarily supportive
        (b)   Rest should be recommended during acute phases
        (c)   Patient should avoid alcohol and substances toxic to liver
        (d)   Full recovery usually within 1 month
        (e)   Patient education should be given advising avoidance of
                unbottled drinking water, ice, shellfish or unpeeled fruits
                and vegetables in endemic areas
        (f)   Hepatitis A vaccine is available prior to deployment to
                endemic areas
(4)   **Hepatitis B and Hepatitis C**- inflammation of the liver caused by a
        Hepatitis B virus or Hepatitis C virus
        (a)   Transmission is parenteral, with the virus found in body
                fluids such as blood, semen and saliva
        (b)   Sexual transmission is common
        (c)   IV drug usage is also and important mode for transmission
(5)   Assessment findings
        (a)   Jaundice
        (b)   Fatigue
        (c)   Nausea and vomiting
        (d)   Low grade fever
        (e)   Pale or clay color
        (f)   Abnormal urine color/dark urine
        (g)   Abdominal pain and enlarged liver
        (h)   In Hepatitis C, many patients are asymptomatic
(6)   Provide care

        (a)   Treatment is primarily supportive. Interferon is used with some success in Hepatitis B and C patients.

        (b)   Bedrest and occasionally hospitalization during the acute phase is necessary

        (c)   Patient should avoid alcohol and substances toxic to liver

        (d)   Patient should be informed of preventative measures
- (i) Hepatitis B vaccination series
- (ii) Condoms if sexually active
- (iii) Test for HIV

(7) **Hepatitis D**

        (a)   Hepatitis D occurs only in association with Hepatitis B infection. Mode of transmission is similar to Hepatitis B

        (b)   May increase severity of disease associated with Hepatitis B

        (c)   Treatment is same as for hepatitis B

(8) **Hepatitis E**

        (a)   Hepatitis E is a food and water-borne disease

        (b)   Associated with epidemics where there is fecally contaminated water

        (c)   Treatment and travel precautions are identical to Hepatitis A

(9) **Hepatitis G-** has recently been identified is patients with Hepatitis that was not Hepatitis C

        (a)   Liver disease has not been proven

        (b)   Signs and symptoms have not yet been characterized

Assess for Human Immunodeficiency Virus (HIV)

A viral infection-

Caused by the human immunodeficiency virus (HIV) that gradually destroys the immune system. Although the virus has been found in all body fluids, only blood, semen and vaginal secretions have been implicated in transmission. There are three known routes of transmission:

(1) Sexual transmission (anal, oral or vaginal)
(2) Blood or blood products (transfusions, infected needles)
(3) Perinatal transmission (in utero, at delivery or through breastfeeding)

History of HIV

(1) Initial case definition was established by CDC in 1982
(2) In 1987 and 1993, case definitions were expanded to include additional illnesses

Body systems affected and potential secondary complications - generally related to opportunistic infections that arise as immune system compromise develops

(1) Nervous system - toxoplasmosis of CNS
(2) Immune system - major site of compromise
(3) Respiratory system - pneumocystis carinii pneumonia
(4) Integumentary system - Kaposi's sarcoma

Health care workers -

(1)   At risk increased when:
   (a)   The exposure involves a large quantity of blood
   (b)   Needle or instrument stick needle size, type (hollow bore versus suture), and depth of penetration
   (c)   The exposure to a patient with a terminal HIV related illness, possibly reflecting a higher viral load in the late course of AIDS
   (d)   Universal precautions not adhered to
(2)   Risk needs to be understood in terms of how the exposure occurred, and what factors were involved
(3)   Potential may appear to be high, but the probability may actually be quite low

Assessment findings- Asymptomatic HIV Infection

(1)   Asymptomatic HIV patients must have had no previous signs or symptoms attributable to HIV infection
(2)   History may be suggestive of an acute mononucleosis or flulike syndrome in the past
(3)   Physical examination of asymptomatic HIV patient is completely normal
(4)   Diagnosis is made with laboratory evidence only

Assessment Findings-

Early Symptomatic HIV Infection
(1)   With disease progression, CD4 lymphocyte counts decrease. There is an increased risk of opportunistic infections
(2)   Signs and symptoms associated with early HIV disease are frequently nonspecific

(a)	Fever (h)			Chronic cough
(b)	Sore throat		(i)	Shortness of breath
(c)	Fatigue		(j)	Oral lesions, ulcers
(d)	Myalgia		(k)	Chronic diarrhea
(e)	Weight loss		(l)	Skin rashes
(f)	Night sweats			
(g)	Lymphadenopathy			

(3)   Diagnosis is made with laboratory evidence and presence of one or more opportunistic infections:
   (a)   Oral candidiasis
   (b)   Generalized wasting
   (c)   Generalized lymphadenopathy
   (d)   Hepatosplenomegaly
   (e)   Severe herpes zoster in a previously healthy person
   (f)   Pneumocystis carinii pneumonia

Assessment Findings-

Late Symptomatic HIV Infection

- (1) Progressive destruction of CD4 cells by the HIV virus places the patient at risk for opportunistic infections, routine infections and malignancies
- (2) Symptoms depend on reactivation of previous illness or exposure to new infections. Commonly seen are:
  - (a) Chronic headaches
  - (b) Seizures
  - (c) Chronic diarrhea
  - (d) Weight loss leading to wasting
  - (e) Chronic fever
  - (f) Visual changes leading to blindness

Provide care

- (1) Treatment of HIV is complex and beyond the scope of the handout
- (2) Isolation is unnecessary, ineffective and unjustified
- (3) Observe BSI when treating an HIV patient
- (4) Psychosocial evaluation of the patient is indicated because of the high incidence of family dysfunction, depression and suicide associated with HIV infection
- (5) Sexual partner notification by Preventive Medicine is essential to prevent transmission
- (6) Consistent use of latex condoms, preferably with nonoxynol-9, a spermicide is recommended to prevent sexual transmission of HIV. Petroleum based lubricants should be avoided because they increase the risk of condom rupture

Assess and Treat for Lyme Disease

An acute inflammatory disease-

Caused by the spirochete Borrelia burgdorferi Transmitted by the bite of a deer tick.

Assessment findings-

- (1) An early localized stage with a painless skin lesion at the site of the bite, called erythema migrans (EM), and a flu-like syndrome with malaise, myalgia
- (2) EM starts off as a red, flat, round rash which spreads out; the outer border remains bright red, with the center becoming clear, blue, or even necrose and turn black
- (3) Incubation period until EM - 3 to 32 days post tick exposure
- (4) Fever and headache
- (5) Inflammation in the knees and other large joints in systemic infection

Patient management and control measures

- (1) The 91W Medic who works, or treats/ transports casualties in a wilderness environment, should be vigilant to the presence of ticks on themselves and their casualties
- (2) There is no evidence of natural transmission from person-to-person
- (3) Tetracycline is the drug of choice given 500mg four times a day for 10-30 days

(4)   Consider anti-inflammatory medications to relieve joint stiffness

Identify Viral Diseases of Childhood

Chickenpox

(1)   A highly contagious, usually mild childhood disease caused by the Herpes varicella-zoster virus.

(2)   Assessment findings
- (a)   Begins with:
  - (i)   Mild respiratory symptoms
  - (ii)   Malaise
  - (iii)   Low-grade fever
- (b)   Rash begins as small red spots that become raised blisters on a red base. These fluid-filled vesicles eventually collapse and dry into scabs
- (c)   Intense itching

(3)   Provide care
- (a)   Do NOT give aspirin due to association with Varicella and Reye's syndrome.
- (b)   Isolation of patient from medical offices, emergency departments, and public places until all lesions are crusted and dry
- (c)   Consider antiviral drugs exist that shortens the duration of symptoms and pain in the older patient
- (d)   Soldier medics who have not had chickenpox should inquire with their chain of command about receiving the chickenpox vaccine
- (e)   VZIG (Varicella Zoster immune globulin) is recommended for pregnant women with a substantial exposure (household contact, close indoor contact > 1 hour, or prolonged direct face-to-face contact with infected person) to chickenpox with no history of previous exposure to chickenpox

Mumps

(1)   An acute, contagious viral disease that causes painful enlargement of the salivary or parotid glands

(2)   Assessment findings
- (a)   Fever
- (b)   Swelling
- (c)   Tenderness of salivary glands, especially parotid
- (d)   Sore throat

(3)   Provide care
- (a)   There is no specific treatment for mumps. Measles, Mumps, Rubella (MMR) immunization should be considered.
- (b)   Symptoms may be relieved by:
  - (i)   Ice or heat to affected neck area
  - (ii)   Acetaminophen for pain relief
  - (iii)   Warm salt water gargles

(iv)   Soft foods
(v)   Extra fluids

Rubella (German Measles)

(1)   A contagious viral infection with mild symptoms associated with a rash
(2)   Assessment findings
      (a)   A rash that spreads from forehead to face to torso to extremities, and lasts 3 days,
      (b)   Serious complications, such as encephalitis, which may occur in measles, do not occur in Rubella
      (c)   Younger females sometimes develop a self-limiting arthritis
      (d)   Cloudy cornea
      (e)   Low grade fever
      (f)   Inflammation of the eyes
(3)   Provide medical care
      (a)   Consider MMR immunization
      (b)   There is no treatment- supportive care primarily
      (c)   Acetaminophen can be given to reduce fever

Measles (rubeola, red measles)

(1)   Highly contagious viral illness
(2)   Assessment findings
      (a)   Conjunctivitis
      (b)   Swelling of the eyelids
      (c)   Photophobia
      (d)   High fevers to 105 degrees
      (e)   Hacking cough
      (f)   Malaise
      (g)   Rash
(3)   Provide care
      (a)   Immunization
          (i)   Effective immunization should be instituted for every person, and is available for combination with other vaccines and/ or toxoids (MMR)
          (ii)   Immunization in children is believed to confer 99% immunogenicity
      (b)   There is no specific treatment. Symptomatic care:
          (i)   Bed rest
          (ii)   Acetaminophen
          (iii)   Humidified air

Pertussis (Whooping cough)

(1)   A highly contagious bacterial disease that affects the respiratory system and produces spasms of coughing that usually end in a high-pitched crowing inspiration (whooping sound)
(2)   Assessment findings

	(a)	Cough
	(b)	Crowing or high-pitched inspiratory whoop
	(c)	Expulsion of clear mucous
	(d)	Vomiting
(3)		Provide care
	(a)	Erythromycin is given 500mg four times a day for 10 days
	(b)	Consider oxygen with high humidity
	(c)	Intravenous fluids may be indicated if coughing is severe enough to prevent adequate oral fluid intake

Reporting an Exposure to an Infectious/ Communicable Disease

What constitutes an exposure?

The following should be considered an exposure incident:
(1)   Eye
(2)   Mouth
(3)   Other mucous membranes
(4)   Non-intact skin
(5)   Parenteral contact with blood
(6)   Blood products
(7)   Other potentially infectious materials

Why it is important to report?

(1)   Permits immediate medical follow up, permitting identification of infection and immediate intervention
(2)   Enables the Designated Officer (DO) to evaluate the circumstances surrounding the incident and implement engineering or procedural changes to avoid a future exposure
(3)   Facilitates follow up testing of the source individual if permission for testing can be obtained
    (a)   Under provisions of the Ryan White Act, the exposed employee has the right to request the infection status of the source casualty from the casualty's health care provider, but neither the agency nor the employee can force testing of the source individual
    (b)   Employers must, and should as part of an effective Exposure Control Plan, tell the employee what to do if an exposure incident occurs

Preventing disease transmission

(1)   Notify supervisor for proper disposition
    (a)   If you have diarrhea
    (b)   If you have a draining wound or any type of wet lesions; wait until lesions are crusted and dry
    (c)   If you are jaundiced
    (d)   If you have been told you have mononucleosis/hepatitis
    (e)   If you have not been treated with a medication and/ or shampoo for lice and scabies
    (f)   Until you have been taking antibiotics for at least 24 hours for a step throat

      (g)   Observe BSI
(i) Always wear gloves
(ii) If chance of splash, wear protective eyewear or face shield
(iii) If large volumes of blood are possibility, wear a gown
(iv) When contacting a possible TB casualty, wear appropriate particulate mask

      (h)   Patients with coughs, headaches, general weakness, recent weight loss, stiff necks, high fevers, and taking medications suggestive of an infectious process are tip-offs in history taking, with experience, the list will get longer for you

      (i)   If after a call with lice, scabies, ticks or other insect vectors
      (i)   Spray the stretcher and casualty compartment with an insecticide, then wipe off/ mop up insecticide residue
      (ii)   Bag the linen separately, and ensure that it not be taken home; bottom line is that it needs to be washed separately
      (iii)   Report any infectious exposure to the designated officer/ manager of your agency identified as such

(2)   Effective hand washing, to include the webs of the hands

(3)   The major infectious diseases that 91W Medic personnel should have in-depth knowledge of for purposes of regulatory compliance
      (a)   HIV
      (b)   Hepatitis
      (c)   Tuberculosis
      (d)   Sexually transmitted diseases

(4)   Understand the concept of occupational risk
      (1)   Appreciate that infectious agent mode of entry, virulence, dose, and host resistance factors combine to define risk, or potential for infection
      (2)   Just because there is risk, doesn't mean that you will become infected
      (3)   Not all infectious diseases are communicable and do not always pose risks to family members
      (4)   Risk and potential does not necessarily equate to probability; HIV is a good example - risks for infection may appear to be high, but the probability of occupational exposure is very low (0.2-0.44%)

Medical and legal aspects of reporting and recording an exposure

(1)   Out-of-hospital personnel deal with very few infectious disease emergencies, but must be vigilant about consequences to themselves, as well as their casualties and coworkers, based on daily, often unknown exposures to infectious agents

(2)   Universal/ standard precautions for soldier medics are superseded by body substance isolation guidelines, based upon the premise that all body fluids, in any situation, may be infectious

(3)   Contact Preventive Medicine for any questions concerning infectious diseases and reporting protocols

Appendix A
Insert and Remove NG Tube
Competency Skill Sheets

NG Tube Insertion

Soldiers Name: _____ SSN: _____ CO: _____ TM: _____
Start: _____ Stop: _____ Initial Evaluator: _____
Start: _____ Stop: _____ Retest Evaluator: _____
Start: _____ Stop: _____ Final Evaluator: _____

		1st	2nd	3rd
a.	Checked doctors orders.	P / F	P / F	P / F
b.	Washed hands. Removed rings and watch.	P / F	P / F	P / F
c.	Gathered and assembled equipment.	P / F	P / F	P / F
d.	Identified patient and explained procedure.	P / F	P / F	P / F
e.	Prepared and positioned patient. (1) Removed dentures, if used. (2) Washed hands. (3) Hyperextended neck. (4) Protected patient with protective pad or towel. (5) Donned gloves.	P / F	P / F	P / F
f.	Measured the tube for insertion distance (Tip of nose-proximal earlobe-tip of sternum). Marked with tape.	P / F	P / F	P / F
g.	Inspected nasal.	P / F	P / F	P / F
h.	Lubricated the tip of NG tube with water soluble lubricant.	P / F	P / F	P / F
i.	Inserted NG tube. (1) Inserted tube into nostril while pointing tip backward and downward. (2) Stopped when first mark on tube is at tip of the nose. (3) Used flashlight to inspect back of throat. (4) Instructed patient to lower chin to chest and swallow sips of water through straw. (5) Advanced tube 3 to 5 inches each time patient swallows. (6) Continued advancing until reach second tape mark.	P / F	P / F	P / F
j.	Checked tube placement.	P / F	P / F	P / F
k.	Anchored tube.	P / F	P / F	P / F
l.	Clamped or connected tube to suction.	P / F	P / F	P / F
m.	Positioned patient with a minimum head elevation of 30 degrees, to prevent gastric reflux.	P / F	P / F	P / F
n.	Removed gloves and washed hands.	P / F	P / F	P / F
o.	Recorded procedure.	P / F	P / F	P / F

Instructor Comments:

NG Removal

Soldiers Name: _____ SSN: _____ CO: _____ TM: _____
Start: _____ Stop: _____ Initial Evaluator: _____
Start: _____ Stop: _____ Retest Evaluator: _____
Start: _____ Stop: _____ Final Evaluator: _____

		1st	2nd	3rd
a.	Identified patient and explained procedure.	P / F	P / F	P / F
b.	Washed hands and donned gloves.	P / F	P / F	P / F
c.	Untapped tube.	P / F	P / F	P / F
d.	Enclosed tube within the towel or glove. Discarded appropriately.	P / F	P / F	P / F
e.	Removed gloves and washed hands.	P / F	P / F	P / F
f.	Instructed patient on mouth care (or provide if necessary).	P / F	P / F	P / F
g.	Encouraged patient to clear nose of mucus and debris.	P / F	P / F	P / F
h.	Documented.	P / F	P / F	P / F

Instructor Comments:

Appendix B
Insert and Remove Foley Catheter
Competency Skill Sheets

Insert Foley Catheter

Soldiers Name: _____ SSN: _____ CO: _____ TM: _____
Start: _____ Stop: _____ Initial Evaluator: _____
Start: _____ Stop: _____ Retest Evaluator: _____
Start: _____ Stop: _____ Final Evaluator: _____

		1st	2nd	3rd
a.	Checked doctor's orders.	P / F	P / F	P / F
b.	Washed hands.	P / F	P / F	P / F
c.	Gathered and assembled equipment.	P / F	P / F	P / F
d.	Identified patient and explained procedure.	P / F	P / F	P / F
e.	Positioned and draped patient.	P / F	P / F	P / F
f.	Opened catheter tray.	P / F	P / F	P / F
g.	Donned sterile gloves.	P / F	P / F	P / F
h.	Positioned moisture-proof pad under patient buttocks (female) (1) Placed moisture-proof pad across upper thighs with fenestrate pad over genitalia (males) (2) Placed fenestrated pad with opening exposing genitalia for females.	P / F	P / F	P / F
i.	Set up sterile field. Prepared equipment and tested balloon.	P / F	P / F	P / F
j.	Cleaned genitalia.	P / F	P / F	P / F
k.	Lubricated catheter.	P / F	P / F	P / F
l.	Inserted catheter until urine flow is observed. Inserted an additional one inch.	P / F	P / F	P / F
m.	Inflated balloon and repositioned catheter.	P / F	P / F	P / F
n.	Hung drainage bag from bed frame.	P / F	P / F	P / F
o.	Removed tray and secured catheter. (1) Taped to thigh of female patient. (2) Taped to abdomen of male patient.	P / F	P / F	P / F
p.	Removed and disposed of gloves. Washed hands.	P / F	P / F	P / F
q.	Recorded procedure.	P / F	P / F	P / F

Instructor Comments:

Remove Foley Catheter

Soldiers Name: _____ SSN: _____ CO: _____ TM:

Start: _____ Stop: _____ Initial Evaluator: _____
Start: _____ Stop: _____ Retest Evaluator: _____
Start: _____ Stop: _____ Final Evaluator: _____

		1st	2nd	3rd
a.	Checked doctor's orders.	P / F	P / F	P / F
b.	Washed hands.	P / F	P / F	P / F
c.	Identified patient and explained procedure.	P / F	P / F	P / F
d.	Positioned and draped patient.	P / F	P / F	P / F
e.	Untaped catheter.	P / F	P / F	P / F
f.	Deflated balloon.	P / F	P / F	P / F
h.	Removed catheter.	P / F	P / F	P / F
i.	Removed equipment and drainage system.	P / F	P / F	P / F
j.	Recorded procedure.	P / F	P / F	P / F

Instructor Comments:

Clinical Handbook

Supportive Care 2

This page intentionally left blank.

91W10
Advanced Individual
Training Course

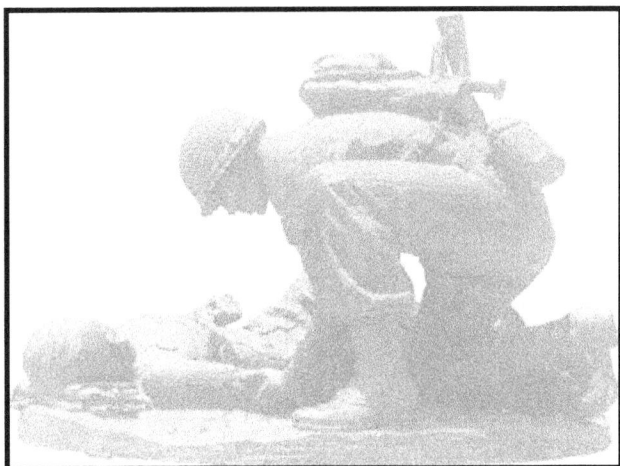

Clinical Handbook
Supportive Care 2

Department of the Army
Academy of Health Sciences
Fort Sam Houston, Texas 78234

TERMINAL LEARNING OBJECTIVE

Given a standard fully stocked M5 Bag or Combat Medic Vest System, given a casualty displaying seizure activity. No other injuries are identified. IAW *Emergency Care in the Streets*, *Prehospital Emergency Care*, *Trauma AIMS*

Types of seizure
  Identify cause of seizure
  (1) Failure to take prescribed anti seizure medication; most common cause of seizures in adults
  (2) Trauma - may occur following head injury (Has the casualty fallen? Has casualty been hit in the head?)
  (3) Congenital brain defect - most often seen in infants and children
  (4) Infection - causes swelling or inflammation of the brain (meningitis or encephalitis)
  (5) Fever - seen in children 6 months to 3 years of age usually with temperatures above 103 degrees; rarely in older children or adults
  (6) Metabolic disorders - irregularities in body chemistry (diabetes/hypoglycemia)
  (7) Drug toxicity - drug/alcohol use or abuse or withdrawal
  (8) Brain tumor - may manifest as a seizure
  (9) Previous trauma - scars on the brain from previous injuries
  (10) Idiopathic - An idiopathic seizure is spontaneous. The cause of the seizure is unknown. It often starts in childhood.
  (11) Hypoxia - lack of oxygen to the brain
  (12) Hypertension - blood pressure is too high; seizures may be associated with cardiovascular accident (CVA)

  Signs and symptoms
  (1) Generalized seizures
       (a) Tonic-clonic seizure (grand mal seizure)
            "Tonic" is muscle tension (stiffness or rigidity).
            "Clonic" is the alternating contraction and relaxation of muscles in rapid succession.

            (i)   May or may not be preceded by an aura
            (ii)   Loss of consciousness occurs
            (iii) Characterized by tonic/clonic seizure activity throughout the entire body
            (iv)   Lasts several minutes (1 to 3)
            (v)   Following by a postictal phase (the patient is confused, drowsy, or unconscious)
            (vi)   Type of seizure that most people associate with epilepsy and other seizure disorders
       (b) Absence seizure (petit mal seizure)
            (i)   Demonstrates temporary loss of awareness to environment
            (ii)   May appear to be daydreaming or staring into space
            (iii) Eyelids may flutter rapidly

1

    (iv)   The person may become unresponsive for a few seconds, then, immediately resume the task he was doing prior to the seizure. The Individual is completely unaware that anything unusual has happened.

    (v)   No tonic or clonic activity

(2) Partial seizures
    (a)   Simple partial seizure (also called Jacksonian seizure)
        (i)   Characterized by tonic and/or clonic movements in only one part of the body
        (ii)   No loss of consciousness
        (iii)   May progress to a generalized seizure
    (b)   Complex partial seizure (also called psychomotor or temporal lobe seizure)
        (i)   Usually preceded by an aura
        (ii)   No loss of consciousness
        (iii)   May be characterized by confusion, glassy stare, aimless movement, fidgeting, lip smacking, and chewing. The person may appear drunk or on drugs.
        (iv)   May progress to a generalized seizure

(3) Status epilepticus
    (a)   Two or more seizures without a period of consciousness between each seizure or a seizure lasting longer than 30 minutes
        (i)   Permanent CNS injury is more likely to occur the longer seizures are allowed to progress
        (ii)   Initiate treatment if continuous seizure activity lasting more than 10 minutes
        (iii)   The longer the seizure is allowed to continue the more difficult it will be to control
        (iv)   Tonic/chonic activity present; may cause long bone and spinal fractures
        (v)   Convulsive activity may gradually lessen over time – giving impression that seizures have been controlled
        (vi)   Correct diagnosis requires a high index of suspicion, a perceptive physician and sometimes an EEG
    (b)   Patient does not have time to breathe well or time to recover between seizures (hypoxia)
    (c)   True medical emergency - receives highest priority for triage and transport in mass casualty situations

Assess the casualty and overview of differential diagnosis
Report a detailed history of the seizure activity
    (1) Physical description
        (a)   Gradual or abrupt onset

     (b)   Progression of motor activity
     (c)   Loss of bowel or bladder control
     (d)   Activity local or generalized
     (e)   Duration of the attack
     (f)   Ask patient if they have any recollection of the attack

(2)   Clinical context of the seizure activity
    (a)   Patient known epileptic
         (i)   Missed doses of antiepileptic or recent alterations in medication
         (ii)   Sleep deprivation
         (iii)   Alcohol withdrawal
         (iv)   Infection
         (v)   Use of other drugs
    (b)   No previous history of seizures
         (i)   Symptoms that might suggest previous unwitnessed or unrecognized seizures
               *   Blank or staring spells in school
               *   Involuntary movements
               *   Unexplained injures
               *   Nocturnal tongue biting
               *   Enuresis
         (ii)   History of recent or remote head injury
         (iii)   Persistent, severe, or sudden headache
         (iv)   Concurrent pregnancy or recent delivery – possible eclampsia
         (v)   History of metabolic derangement or electrolyte abnormalities, hypoxia, systemic illness (especially cancer), coagulopathy or anticoagulation, drug ingestion or withdrawal and alcohol use

General physical examination
Is directed toward discovering any injuries, especially to the head or spine, resulting from seizure.
(1)   Possible fractures, sprains and bruises
(2)   Tongue lacerations
(3)   Assess for precipitating factors. Search for any systemic illness that may have caused the seizure.
(4)   Assess vital signs, note temperature
(5)   Assess blood glucose level, if equipment available
(6)   Assess for motor system coordination, strength and tone
(7)   Assess for slurred, very weak or hoarse speech
(8)   Assess for jerky, uncoordinated, slumped or slow movements in posture and gait
(9)   Assess for incontinence of bladder and bowel

Differential Diagnosis
Many episodic disturbances of neurologic function may be mistaken for seizures.

The following are several of the more important entities that should be considered.

Syncope
(a)	Symptoms: may include some or all of the following: dizziness, diaphoresis, nausea, and "tunnel vision"
(b)	Patient is usually aware they are going to faint
(c)	Can describe onset of attack
(d)	Cardiac Syncope may occur suddenly without any warning
(e)	Injury or incontinence may occur

Pseudoseizures (extremely difficult to distinguish from true seizures)
(a)	Pseudoseizures are psychiatric rather than neurogenic
(b)	Associated with conversion disorder, panic disorder, psychosis, and impulse control disorder
(c)	May occur in response to emotional upset
(d)	Attack will occur with witnesses present
(e)	Incontinence, injury, postictal confusion and lethargy are uncommon

Hyperventilation syndrome
(a)	Gradual onset
(b)	Shortness of breath, anxiety, and perioral numbness
(c)	May progress to involuntary spasm or the extremities and even loss of consciousness

Migraines
(a)	Similar to aura of partial seizures

Movement disorders
(a)	Dystonia, chorea, myoclonic jerks, tremors, or tics may occur in a variety of neurologic conditions
(b)	Consciousness is always preserved during movements
(d)	Involuntary but can be suppressed by patient

Clinical features that help to distinguish seizures from other kinds of mimicking attacks include:
(a)	Abrupt onset and termination
(b)	Lack of recall
(c)	Movements of behavior during the attack generally are purposeless or inappropriate
(d)	Attack is followed by a period of postictal confusion and lethargy (except for petit mal or simple partial seizures)

4

Provide emergency medical care
Treatment
During a seizure
    (a)   Position the patient on the floor or the ground. Move the furniture with edges away from the patient (GOAL: prevent self-injury)

    (b)   DO NOT RESTRAIN the patient during a seizure

    (c)   DO NOT force anything into the patient's mouth

WARNING: Bite sticks have been bitten and swallowed resulting in an airway obstruction. Teeth and jaws have been broken due to forcing a tongue blade into the mouth. NEVER use fingers to keep the patient's teeth apart.

    (d)   Observe and record time of onset, duration, characteristics of the seizure, and if the patient was incontinent of stool or urine

CAUTION: If the casualty's teeth are clenched, do not attempt to forcibly open the casualty's jaw. Do not restrain the casualty's limbs during seizures.

After a seizure
    (a)   Maintain an open airway
        (i)   Position casualty to maintain open airway
        (ii)   Clear airway
        (iii)   Insert airway device to assist with maintaining open airway, if needed
        (iv)   Support and stabilize cervical spine, if suspected injury

    (b)   Turn patient on his side if no spinal trauma is suspected and suction his mouth as needed

    (c)   Administer high-flow oxygen. Use a non-rebreather mask if the patient is breathing on his own. Use BVM with reservoir to ventilate if patient is NOT breathing on his own.

    (d)   Monitor vital signs

    (e)   Protect the patient from embarrassment. Cover the patient if exposed or clothes are torn. Keep spectators away from area. If patient loses bladder/bowel control, clean and/or cover the patient as soon as possible.

    (f)   Establish and maintain intravenous access

    (g)   Administer IV fluids cautiously

Administer pharmacological interventions
    (a)   Valium
        (i)   Therapeutic effects
            *   Suppress seizure activity in the motor cortex of the brain

        *   Generalized central nervous system depressant

        *   Muscle relaxant

(ii)   Indications

        *   To treat grand mal seizures/status epilepticus/seizures lasting greater than 10 to 15 minutes

(iii)   Contraindications

        *   Should not be given during pregnancy - exception may be seizures associated with eclampsia

        *   Should not be given to patients with hypotension/decreased systolic BP less than 90

        *   Should not be given to patients with respiratory depression. Respiration less than 10 per minute

(iv)   Side effect

        *   Possible hypotension

        *   Depression in the level of consciousness

(v)   Administration and dosage

        *   For grand mal seizures/status epilepticus give slow IV in titrated doses. Can be given intramuscular, rectally, or via endotracheal tube if needed. Start with 2.5 mg. Monitor vital signs. If vital signs are stable and patient is still seizing, give another 2.5 mg of Valium slow IV push. Continue until the seizures have stopped. Do not exceed total dosage of 10 mg.

(vi)   Incompatibility

        *   Should not be mixed with any other drug

(b)   50% Dextrose (D50)

    (i)   Therapeutic effects

        *   Rapidly restores blood sugar level to normal level

    (ii)   Indications

        *   To treat suspected hypoglycemia

        *   To treat status epilepticus

    (iii)   Contraindications

        *   Intracranial hemorrhage

        *   Known stroke

    (iv)   Side effects

        *   Will cause tissue necrosis if it infiltrates

              *   May precipitate severe neurological symptoms in alcoholics (Wernieke's Encephalopathy)

(v)   Administration and dosage
        *   50 ml of 50% solution (25 gm) slow IV. Supplied in pre-filled syringes containing 50 ml of 50% solution.
        *   Determine serum glucose if possible prior to administering glucose

(c)   Ativan (Lorazepam)

    (i)   Indications
        *   Anxiety disturbances or anxiety states: general anxiety disturbances panic disturbances phobic anxiety disturbances
        *   Adjustment disturbances with anxiety or stress reaction

    (ii)   Contraindications
        *   Assess patient periodically
        *   Safety and efficacy in children under the age of 12 has not been established

    (iii)   Dosages
        *   ADULT dose for anxiety is: 2mg - 3mg daily in 3 - 4 divided doses
        *   RANGE: 1mg - 6mg daily in divided doses
        *   ELDERLY/DEBILITATED PATIENTS: Initial dose of 1mg - 2mg/day in divided doses. Adjust as needed and tolerated.
        *   In elderly and/or debilitated patients and in those with serious respiratory or cardiovascular disease, a reduction in dosage is recommended
        *   In the case of local anesthesia and diagnostic procedures requiring patient co-operation, concomitant use of an analgesic is recommended.
        *   Ativan sl: Dosage of ativan sublingual should be individualized for maximum effect.

CAUTION: The soldier medic must be proficient and competent in drug administration. This includes knowledge of therapeutic effect, indications, contraindications, side effects, how supplied, administration, and dosage of the drugs.

    (d)   After the seizure activity is over, assess and treat any injuries suffered during the seizure

(e) Expect lethargy, partial consciousness, and disorientation
(f) If possible, try to determine how long the seizure lasted, what the patient did after the seizure, and what the patient was doing prior to the seizure

Transport considerations
Requirements
(a) Patient with a first time or new seizure
(b) Patient with a seizure that caused injury
(c) Patient with respiratory difficulty
(d) Status epilepticus patient - immediate transport
Maintain an open airway
Patient should be transported on his side while being given supplemental oxygen en route to the medical facility
Suction mouth as needed
Monitor vital signs while en route

Provide on-going management
Maintain the casualty on their side, if necessary
Monitor the casualty's airway
Monitor vital signs to include pulse oximetry, if available
Monitor neurological status
(1) Pupil response
(2) Glasgow coma scale
   (a) Eye opening
   (b) Verbal response
   (c) Motor response
Place the casualty in a quiet, reassuring environment, if possible
Monitor IV fluids.
Reassess pharmacological interventions every 15-30 min.

CAUTION: Sudden, loud noises or bright light may cause another seizure

Document seizure activity
(1) Duration of the seizure
(2) Presence of cyanosis, breathing difficulty, or apnea
(3) Level of consciousness before, during and after the seizure
(4) Preceded by aura (ask the casualty)
(5) Muscles involved (type of motor activity)
(6) Incontinence of bladder or bowel
(7) Eye movement
(8) Previous history of seizures, head trauma, and/or drug or alcohol abuse

Evacuate the casualty by ground, if possible

TERMINAL LEARNING OBJECTIVE

Given a standard fully stocked M5 Bag or Combat Medic Vest System, with an obstetric kit. You encounter a pregnant female who is in labor. IAW *The Basic EMT Comprehensive Prehospital Patient Care*, *EMT Prehospital Care*

Stages of Labor
First stage
(1)   Begins with the onset of regular contractions
    (a)   Contraction time - the span of time from the beginning of a contraction of the uterus to when the uterus relaxes
    (b)   Interval time - the span of time from start of one contraction to the start of the next contraction
(2)   Rupture of amniotic sac

WARNING: "Meconium staining" - amniotic fluid that is greenish or brownish-yellow rather than clear, is an indication of possible fetal distress during labor.

(3)   Appearance of bloody show

(4)   Ends with the full dilation and effacement of the cervix

NOTE: In order for a vaginal delivery to occur, the cervix must both thin out (efface) to 100% and open up (dilate) to 10cm (3-4 inches).

WARNING: There is usually time to transport the patient before delivery during this phase.

Second stage
(1)   Begins when the baby enters the birth canal

(2)   Contractions become stronger

(3)   Presenting part appears

(4)   Ends with the birth of the baby

CAUTION: Transportation of the patient at this time should NOT BE CONSIDERED. Delivery is imminent.

Third stage
(1)   Begins when delivery of baby is complete

(2)   Ends with the delivery of the placenta and umbilical cord

Care for Normal Delivery Outside the Hospital
Evaluation of the mother

(1)   Ask the mother the following questions

       (a)   How long have you been pregnant or expected due date?
       (b)   How long and how often she has been having contractions?
       (c)   If she has had any bleeding or bloody show?

(2)   Check for signs and symptoms that indicate delivery will occur before transport is possible

       (a)   Head or other presenting part is visible (crowning)
       (b)   Mother tells you "The baby is coming", especially if she is a multiparous woman
       (c)   Mother feels as if she is having a bowel movement with increasing pressure in the vaginal area
       (d)   Mother feels the need to push
       (e)   Hospital is not accessible due to traffic or weather/disaster
       (f)   Transportation will not become available before anticipated time of delivery

(3)   If delivery is eminent with crowning, contact medical officer for decision to commit to delivery on site. If delivery does not occur within 10 minutes, contact medical officer for permission to transport.

Predelivery preparation of the mother

(1)   Ensure the mother's privacy

(2)   Obtain and open emergency obstetric pack. This will provide all the sterile supplies needed for care of the mother and infant before and after delivery.

(3)   In absence of an emergency obstetric pack medic should collect clean sheets and towels, heavy sting or cord (shoelaces) to tie the cord, a towel or plastic bag to wrap the placenta, and clean unused rubber gloves and eyewear

(4)   Put on gloves, mask, gown, and goggles for infection control precaution if the conditions permit/as time allows

(5)   Position the mother and prepare work space for both delivery and care of the newborn

       (a)   Position mother lying with knees drawn up and spread apart. Elevate the hips with a folded blanket or pillow.
       (b)   Create a sterile field around vaginal opening with sterile towels or paper barriers
       (c)   Have another individual monitoring the airway, render assistance if she should vomit, and provide emotional support

Assist in delivery of the baby

Encourage mother to breathe deeply through her mouth. She may feel better if she pants.

When the infant's head appears during crowning, place fingers on the bony part of skull and exert slight pressure to prevent an explosive delivery. Use caution to avoid "soft spot" (fontanelle.)

If the amniotic sac does not break, or has not broken, use a clamp or your finger to puncture the sac and push it away from the infant's head and mouth as they appear

As the infant's head is being born, determine if the umbilical cord is around the infant's neck
(a)   If the umbilical cord is around the infant's neck, slip it over the shoulder or clamp, cut, and unwrap
(b)   Umbilical cord must be clamped and cut if it is wrapped too tightly around the infant's neck

After the infant's head is born, support the head, suction the mouth first then the nostrils two or three times with a bulb syringe if available

CAUTION: Use caution to avoid contact with the back of the mouth.

(a)   Squeeze the bulb syringe before placing it in the mouth or nose
(b)   Slowly release with withdrawal
(c)   Squeeze again to expel contents before reinserting

Continue to support the baby's head between contractions while waiting for the rest of the body to be delivered

WARNING: DO NOT pull on the baby's head to assist with the delivery.

As the feet are born, grasp the feet. Wipe blood and mucus from mouth and nose again.

Wrap the infant in a warm blanket and place on his side, with the head slightly lower than the trunk

WARNING: Keep infant warm to prevent hypothermia, which can occur quickly.

Keep infant level with vagina until the cord is cut

Have your partner monitor and complete initial care of the newborn

The infant must be breathing on its own before clamping and cutting the cord, palpate the cord with your fingers to make sure it is no longer pulsating
(a)   Use clamps or umbilical tape found in the obstetric kit
(b)   Apply the first clamp about 8 to 10 inches from the baby
(c)   Place the second clamp 2 to 3 inches below the first, approximately 4 fingers width from infant
(d)   Cut the cord between the clamps or knots using sterile surgical scissors

CAUTION: NEVER unclasp a cord once it has been cut, or attempt to adjust a clamp once it is in place.

Observe for delivery of the placenta while preparing mother and infant for transport

When the placenta is delivered, wrap it in a towel and put it in a plastic bag

Place sterile pad over vaginal opening, lower mother's legs, help her hold them together. Transport mother, infant, and placenta to hospital.

Record the birth
  (a)   Document exact time of birth on the run sheet
  (b)   Make a double-backed tape bracelet with the time of birth and the mother's full name. Apply to baby's wrist or ankle.

Caring for the newborn
Position, dry, wipe and wrap the newborn in a blanket and cover the head
  (a)   Place baby in a head-down position
  (b)   Repeat suctioning the mouth and nose as necessary

Assessment of infant - normal findings
  (a)   The APGAR score may be used to evaluate the newborn's condition. Perform as soon as the infant's born and 5 minutes later.
  (b)   Evaluating the adequacy of a newborn's vital functions immediately after birth
  (c)   Five parameters: heart rate, respiratory effort, muscle tone, reflex irritability, and color
  (d)   Each parameter is given a score from 0 to 2
  (e)   Majority of infants are vigorous and have a total score of 7 to 10
         Appearance - note the infant's color. Normal color is pink with some cyanosis of the extremities.

         Pulse - determine the infant's pulse rate. The pulse rate should be greater than 100 per minute.

         Grimace - evaluate the infant's response to an irritable stimulus. The infant should cry or react vigorously.

         Activity - how much is the infant moving? Infant should have good motion in extremities.

         Respiration effort (breathing) - the infant should be breathing within 30 seconds after birth (breathing normal or crying)

Stimulate newborn if not breathing

    (a)   A gentle vigorous rubbing of the baby's back should stimulate breathing, if that fails, snap your index finger against the sole of the feet

    (b)   DO NOT hold the baby upside down to slap its bottom

Resuscitation of the newborn - after assessment, if signs and symptoms require either cardiac or pulmonary resuscitation, perform the following steps when appropriate

    (a)   If breathing effort is shallow, slow, or absent, provide artificial ventilations

        (i)   40 to 60 per minute

        (ii)   Reassess after 30 seconds

        (iii)   If no improvement, continue artificial ventilation and reassessments

    (b)   If heart rate is less than 100 beats per minute, provide artificial ventilations

        (i)   40 to 60 per minute

        (ii)   Reassess after 30 seconds

        (iii)   If no improvement, continue artificial ventilation and reassessments

    (c)   If heart rate is less than 80 beats per minute and not responding to artificial ventilations, start chest compressions

    (d)   If heart rate is less than 60 beats per minute, start compressions and artificial ventilations

        (i)   Chest compressions in the newborn should be delivered at a rate of 120 per minute, mid sternum

        (ii)   Give compressions with two thumbs, fingers supporting the back, at a depth of 1/2 to 3/4 inch

CAUTION: This is for newborns only.

    (e)   Color - if the infant exhibits cyanosis of the face and/or torso with spontaneous breathing and adequate heart rate. Administer oxygen 10 to 15LPM using oxygen tubing held as close as possible, but not directly into the infant's face.

Delivering the placenta
The placenta is normally expelled within minutes after the baby is born. Never pull on the cord to facilitate delivery.

Save the placenta in a container and place it in a plastic bag, or wrap it in a towel or paper and bring it with the mother and baby to the hospital

Emergency care of mother post-delivery - place baby to mothers breast
Up to 500cc if blood loss is normal and well tolerated by the mother following delivery

The soldier medic must be aware of this loss so as not to cause undue psychological stress on him or the new mother

If there is excessive blood loss, massage the uterus
    (a)   Place fully extended fingers on lower abdomen above pubis and massage lightly with a circular motion over area
    (b)   If bleeding continues, check massage technique and transport immediately. Provide oxygen and perform ongoing assessment.

Regardless of estimated blood loss, if mother shows signs and symptoms of shock, treat as such and transport prior to uterine massage. Massage the uterine fundus en route to the hospital.

Monitor for complications during labor
Terms and definitions
Breech birth - delivery with the buttocks, feet, or knees appearing as the presenting part

Premature infant - an infant weighing less than 5.5 lbs. or born before the 37th week of gestation

Meconium - a greenish-black to light brown, material that collects in the intestine of a fetus and forms the first stool of a newborn

Abnormal deliveries of childbirth
Premature infants ("Preemie")
    (a)   Description
            (i)   An infant weighing less than 5.5 lbs. or born before the 37th week of gestation
            (ii)   Smaller and thinner than a full-term baby
            (iii)   The proportion of the head to the body is greater than a full-term infant
    (b)   Treatment and transport - same as for normal births
            (i)   Dry the baby thoroughly as soon as possible after birth
            (ii)   Keep warm - absence of fully developed layer of fatty tissue allows rapid cooling and development of hypothermia
                  *   Wrap completely, with face exposed
                  *   Maintain temperature of room or ambulance at 90-100°
            (iii)   Keep mouth and nose clear of mucus by suctioning frequently
            (iv)   Provide ventilations and/or chest compressions based upon the baby's pulse and respiratory effort (see Annex F)
            (v)   Administer oxygen (humidified, if possible) by directing flow into an improvised tent over baby's face

(vi)   Watch the umbilical cord for bleeding. Apply
         another clamp or tie closer to the abdomen to
         prevent excessive blood loss.
(vii)   Prevent contamination. Wear a gown/mask.
         Keep bystanders at a distance.
(viii)   Handle gently while providing all care
(ix)   Inform hospital of premature delivery

Breech presentation
(a)   Description
      (i)   Presenting part is the buttocks or feet
      (ii)   Most common abnormal delivery
(b)   Treatment and transport
      (i)   Initiate rapid transport upon recognition of a
              breech presentation
      (ii)   Never attempt to deliver the baby by pulling on
              its legs
      (iii)   Provide high concentrations of oxygen
      (iv)   Place the mother in a head-down position with
              the pelvis elevated
      (v)   If the body delivers, support buttocks and trunk
              and prevent an explosive delivery of the head
      (vi)   After delivery, care for the newborn, cord,
              mother, and placenta as in normal delivery.

Prolapsed umbilical cord - a true emergency
(a)   Description
      (i)   Umbilical cord presents first
      (ii)   Oxygen supply to baby is interrupted when the
              cord is squeezed between the vaginal wall and
              the presenting part
      (iii)   Commonly seen with breech deliveries or small
              babies (premature births/multiple births)
(b)   Treatment and transport
      (i)   Perform initial assessment
      (ii)   Place mother with her head down and elevate
              her hips with a blanket or pillow, this will lessen
              pressure on the birth canal
      (iii)   Provide a high concentration of oxygen
      (iv)   Gently push on the presenting part to keep
              pressure off cord, by inserting several fingers of
              your gloved hand into the vagina. Maintain this
              position until relieved by the physician at the
              medical treatment facility.
      (v)   Check the cord for pulses and keep it warm with
              a towel moistened with sterile saline and
              wrapped again with a dry towel
      (vi)   DO NOT attempt to push the cord back inside
              the mother
      (vii)   Transport immediately to a medical facility

       (viii)   Have your partner obtain baseline vital signs, AMPLE history, and physical exam en route to the hospital, if possible

Limb presentation
- (a) Description - arm or leg presents first
- (b) Foot is the most common in a breach presentation
- (c) Limb presentation cannot be delivered in the prehospital setting
- (d) Treatment and transport
  - (i) Place mother in a head down position with hips elevated
  - (ii) Administer a high concentration of oxygen
  - (iii) DO NOT attempt to place the limb back into the vagina
  - (iv) Transport immediately to a medical facility

Multiple birth
- (a) Description - more than one infant is being born (e.g., twins, triplets)
- (b) Treatment and transport
  - (i) Assist as in a single delivery
  - (ii) Clamp and cut the cord of first baby
  - (iii) Note time of first birth
  - (iv) Assist with subsequent births, cut and clamp each cord. Note the time of each birth.
  - (v) Make certain to identify each child and order of birth (1 and 2 or A and B)
  - (vi) Provide care for each infant, mother, umbilical cord, and placenta as with a single delivery

Meconium staining
- (a) Description
  - (i) Greenish or brownish-yellow amniotic fluid. A result of fecal material released from the baby's bowels before birth.
  - (ii) Occurs when the infant is distressed due to cord compression, trauma, or other complications while inside the amniotic sac

CAUTION: Appearance of meconium in amniotic fluid is a sign that the infant has a potentially serious problem. Aspiration of meconium by the infant during delivery can cause severe respiratory complications.

- (b) Treatment and transport
  - (i) Suction the baby's mouth, then nose BEFORE stimulating the baby to breathe. This is to avoid aspiration of amniotic fluid with meconium particles.

(ii)   Continue to monitor the airway
(iii)   Transport immediately
(iv)   Notify hospital of the presence of meconium in the fluid

Predelivery Emergencies

Miscarriage/spontaneous abortion

Fetus and placenta may deliver before the 20th week of pregnancy

(a)   Signs and symptoms
    (i)   Moderate to severe vaginal bleeding
    (ii)   Abnormal cramping
    (iii)   Discharge of tissue, blood, and/or blood clots from the vagina

(b)   Emergency care steps
    (i)   Perform initial assessment
    (ii)   Obtain AMPLE history and baseline vital signs
    (iii)   Initiate and maintain IV with Normal Saline
    (iv)   Treat for shock if indicated
    (v)   Administer high concentration oxygen
    (vi)   Place sanitary pad over the vagina. Save all used pads.
    (vii)   Save all expelled tissue
    (viii)   Provide emotional support
    (ix)   Transport immediately

Ectopic Pregnancy

(a)   95% of all ectopic pregnancies occurs in a fallopian tube

(b)   Usually referred to as a „tubal pregnancy"

(c)   Most likely to occur when the fallopian tube is scarred from infection (PID) or previous abdominal/gynecological surgeries

(d)   Signs and symptoms
    (i)   Abdominal pain initially localized to one side or the other of the lower abdomen
    (ii)   Initially pain is "crampy" and intermittent in nature
    (iii)   As pregnancy progresses, the fallopian tube ruptures and pain becomes constant and diffuse throughout the abdomen
    (iv)   Patient may experience shoulder pain which suggests a large hemoperitoneum
    (v)   Patient may or may not have vaginal bleeding
    (vi)   Patient usually has a history of amenorrhea

(e)   Emergency care and treatment
    (i)   Maintain airway

(ii)   Administer oxygen

(iii)   Keep patient supine

(iv)   Initiate a large bore IV and administer IV fluids

(v)   Keep NPO (nothing by mouth)

(vi)   Transport immediately to definitive care facility

Pre-eclampsia (toxemia of pregnancy)
- (a)   Signs and symptoms
  - (i)   Hypertension
  - (ii)   Proteinuria - protein in the urine
  - (iii)   Elevated blood pressure
  - (iv)   Excessive weight gain
  - (v)   Swelling (edema) of the face, hands, ankles, and feet
- (b)   Emergency care steps
  - (i)   Notify medical officer immediately
  - (ii)   Perform initial assessment
  - (iii)   Obtain SAMPLE history and baseline vital signs
  - (iv)   Treatment based on signs and symptoms
  - (v)   Transport patient on her left side

Eclampsia
- (a)   Signs and Symptoms
  - (i)   Headaches
  - (ii)   Visual disturbances
  - (iii)   Epigastric pain
  - (iv)   Massive swelling (edema) especially of the face and hands
  - (v)   Proteinuria (protein in the urine)
  - (vi)   Seizures - occurrence of seizures clearly marks transition of pre-eclampsia to eclampsia
- (b)   Emergency care and treatment
  - (i)   Position on left side. Keep patient quiet and in a darkened room, if possible
  - (ii)   Administer high flow oxygen
  - (iii)   Initiate and maintain intravenous line
  - (iv)   Transport to hospital as gently and quickly as possible
  - (v)   Anticipate seizure activity. Have suction readily available.
  - (vi)   Pharmacological interventions as directed by MD/PA

Ante partum Hemorrhage (bleeding before delivery)
- (a)   Three main causes
  - (i)   Abruptio placenta - premature separation of the placenta from the wall of the uterus during the last trimester of pregnancy. Patient will experience sudden onset of severe abdominal

pain with or without vaginal bleeding. Fetal movement/fetal heart tones are usually absent. The abdomen will be tender and the uterus rigid to palpation.

    (ii)   Placenta previa - painless vaginal bleeding. Usually bright red. Occurs as the cervix begins to dilate in preparation for delivery and the placenta covers all or part of the cervical canal. Fetal movement continues and fetal heart tones are audible. Uterus is soft and non-tender.

    (iii)   Uterine rupture - usually occurs during labor. Women at risk are multiparous or have had a previous c-section. Vaginal bleeding may or may not be present. Contractions will have lessened or stopped. Patient will exhibit obvious signs of shock.

(b)   Emergency care and management

    (i)   Regardless of cause of third trimester bleeding, management and treatment are the same.

    (ii)   Position on left side

    (iii)   Administer high flow oxygen

    (iv)   Initiate and maintain at least two large-bore IV's

    (v)   Treat for shock

    (vi)   Notify MD/PA Immediately

    (vii)   Evacuate/transport to definitive care facility

Trauma in pregnancy

(a)   Three major causes

    (i)   Motor vehicle crashes

    (ii)   Falls

    (iii)   Penetrating injuries (i.e. gun shot wounds)

(b)   Anatomic changes of pregnancy

    (i)   Compression of abdominal contents into upper abdomen results in a higher incidence of abdominal trauma in association with chest trauma

    (ii)   Bladder is displaced upward and forward so it is outside the pelvic cavity and is at increased risk for injury

    (iii)   The obviously enlarged uterus is at risk for injury/rupture

(c)   Physiologic changes of pregnancy

    (i)   Vascular volume increases to support the perfusion of two circulations (patient and fetus)

    (ii)   Increase in cardiac output to pump increased volume - resting heart rate increases to 15-20 BPM's

    (iii)   Redistribution of blood volume with as much as a tenfold increase in blood flow to the pelvic region

            (iv)   Respiratory changes include an increased need for oxygen due to a higher basal metabolism - increased minute volume

            (v)   Tidal volume increases along with minute volume to rid the body of the increased CO_2 from the patient and fetus

            (vi)   All of the physiologic changes make it difficult to assess for signs and symptoms of shock and to adequately ventilate the patient

(d)   Emergency care and management

            (i)   Treat the mother first

            (ii)   Maintain adequate airway

            (iii)   Administer high flow 02 - oxygen needs are 10 - 20% higher than normal

            (iv)   Assist with ventilations as needed - remember to provide higher minute volume

            (v)   Control external bleeding

            (vi)   Position on left side - lying on the left side will shift the weight of gravid (pregnant) uterus off the vena cava. If immobilized on backboard, tilt board 30 degrees to the left.

            (vii)   Initiate and maintain IV

            (viii)   Transport/evacuate to definitive care facility

Identify additional gynecological emergencies
Ectopic pregnancy

(1)   Assessment findings

      (a)   Acute abdominal pain

      (b)   Vaginal bleeding

      (c)   Rapid and weak pulse

      (d)   Low blood pressure

(2)   Notify MD/PA

(3)   Prepare for immediate transport

(4)   Maintain ABC's

(5)   Administer high flow 02

(6)   Initiate and maintain IV with Normal Saline

(7)   Reassess continuously

TERMINAL LEARNING OBJECTIVE

Given a patient medical record, immunization record, supplies, and equipment at Echelon II and below, provide soldier readiness processing for a company size element. Evaluate a patient who presents for an Ambulatory Medical Visit (Sick Call). Performed soldier readiness processing in support of unit deployment. Evaluated a patient who presents for an Ambulatory Medical Visit.

Screen medical records for accuracy and completeness

> **Primary goal of the medical screener is to provide timely, quality care for active duty personnel with minor medical conditions**
> (1)   Do not function as independent providers
> (2)   Work under the direct supervision of a medical officer who is responsible for the care the medic provides
>
> **The following guidelines must be followed:**
> (1)   The SOAP format must be used when evaluating a patient
> (2)   Consult with the supervising medical officer prior to the patient leaving the treatment facility
> (3)   Know your limitations and immediately refer to an MD/PA any patient with one of the following conditions:
>> (a)   Febrile illness with temperature exceeding 101° F
>> (b)   Acute distress such as, breathing difficulties, chest pain, acute abdominal pain, suspected fractures, lacerations, etc.
>> (c)   Altered mental status
>> (d)   Unexplained pulse above 120 per minute
>> (e)   Unexplained respiratory rate above 24 or less then 8 per minute
>> (f)   Diastolic blood pressure over 100 mm Hg systolic BP less than 90 mmHg
>
> **Soldier medic's responsibilities during medical screening procedures (sick call)**
> (1)   Validate identification of soldier
> (2)   Gather sick slip and review
> (3)   Sign patient in and pull soldier's medical record (Initiate a replacement record if required)
> (4)   Complete vital signs and document on appropriate form (e.g. DA Form 5181, SF 600, and DD Form 689
> (5)   Check for medical profile(s) (temporary or permanent)
> (6)   Check Over 40 Physical (as required)
> (7)   Check for eyeglasses and protective mask inserts (as required)
> (8)   Check for DNA sample
> (9)   Check for Medical Warning Tags (DA Form 3365)
> (10)   Refer to medical authority as required
> (11)   Screen individual IAW APC, Algorithm-Directed Troop Medical Care, HSC Pam 40-7-21, for soldier's chief complaint

(12)   Follow algorithm protocol for disposition and/or treatment and
         annotate on appropriate form
(13)   Sign individual out of BAS and follow appropriate disposition after
         screened by medic or PA evaluation
(14)   Clean and set up screening area for next individual reporting to sick
         call
(15)   Secure medical record

Screen immunization records for accuracy and completeness

Screen immunization records
(1)   Validate identification of soldier
(2)   Ensure all immunizations are current on PHS 731 (Shot Record)
        (a)   Refer to medical record if shot record is not available
        (b)   Inquire regarding allergic reactions
        (c)   Check for Medical Warning Tags
        (d)   Refer to immunization site if immunizations are required
(3)   Return immunization record to soldier
(4)   Secure medical record

Shot Call
(1)   Persons who administer vaccinations must be trained in:
        (a)   Management of anaphylaxis
        (b)   Immunization procedures
        (b)   Proper use and maintenance of equipment
        (c)   Indications and contraindications for each vaccine
        (d)   Storage requirements
        (e)   Management and reporting of adverse reactions
        (f)   Immunization record maintenance
(2)   Patients who report to shot call should be:
        (a)   Screened for chronic/acute illness
        (b)   Screened for pregnancy
        (c)   Screened for medications that might interact with
                immunizations
        (d)   Screened for allergies
        (e)   Offer Tylenol to minimize local and systemic shot reactions
        (f)   Observed for at least 20 minutes after administration for
                symptoms of anaphylaxis

Screen for personnel / administrative matters

S-1 personnel (administration) center will screen these records

Validate / inspect Identification Card (DD Form 2A)

**Validate / inspect Geneva Conventions ID Card (DD Form 1934)(as
required)**

Refer for new card(s) as required

Check Identification tags (2 sets) for accuracy

Screen Dental Records

Review date of last dental examination
(1)   Ensure Class 1 or 2
(2)   Ensure Dental X-rays (Panorex) is present and up to date

Refer to Dental authority as required

Ask and record the following Medical History information on the prescribed form

Purpose of the Chronological Medical Record
(1)   To improve communication among all those caring for the patient
(2)   To display the assessment, problems and plans in an organized format to facilitate the care of the patient and for use in record review and quality control

Ask and record medical history information
(1)   Identifying data
(2)   Chief complaint:
        (a)   Concise statement
        (b)   Primary reason the patient seeks help
        (c)   Use patient's own words
(3)   Present illness:
        (a)   State of health prior to onset of illness
        (b)   Nature and circumstances of onset
        (c)   Location and nature of pain or discomfort
        (d)   Progression
        (e)   Treatment received and its effect
(4)   Past history:
        (a)   Childhood diseases
        (b)   Previous illnesses and injuries
        (c)   Previous hospitalization and surgery
(5)   Family history:
        (a)   History of chronic illness
        (b)   Familial illness (sickle cell)
(6)   Social history:
        (a)   Marital status
        (b)   Occupational data
        (c)   Habits (tobacco, alcohol, drugs)

Use the SOAP Note Format
(1)   **S:** SUBJECTIVE DATA: what the patient tells you
(2)   **O:** OBJECTIVE - physical findings and lab/ X-ray
(3)   **A.:** ASSESSMENT - Your interpretation of the patient's condition
(4)   **P:** PLAN

Perform a patient examination

Determine what is wrong with the patient based on patient's own statements regarding his specific condition.

Determine the chief complaint based on the patient's own statements: Focused examination based on chief complaint

The S.O.A.P. (E. R.) method is the only accepted method of medical record entries for the military
(1)   **S:** (subjective) - What the patient tells you
(2)   **O:** (objective) - Physical findings of the exam
(3)   **A:** (assessment) - Your interpretation of the patients condition
(4)   **P:** (plan) - Includes the following
    (a)   Therapeutic treatment: includes use of meds, use of bandages, etc.
    (b)   Additional diagnostic procedures: any test that still might be needed
(5)   **E:** (patient education) - special instructions, handouts, use of medications, side effects, etc.
(6)   **R:** (return to clinic) - when and under what circumstances to return.

Components of the patient examination (SOAP note)
(1)   Medical History - Gives you an idea of the patient's problem before you start physical exam
    (a)   Biographic data
    (b)   Chief complaint
        (i)   This is the reason for the patients visit
        (ii)   Use direct quotes from patient
        (iii)   Avoid diagnostic terms
    (c)   Observation: begins as soon as the patient walks through the door
    (d)   Listening: listen carefully. This will help you get an accurate diagnosis of the problem
    (e)   Open ended questions: help you to get more complete and accurate information
    (f)   Provider obstacles: your attitude or predetermination may prevent you from making an accurate judgment
    (g)   Patient obstacles: the patient has many obstacles to overcome. Patients must have confidence in you.
(2)   History of present illness/injury (HPI)
    (a)   Duration: when the illness/injury started
    (b)   Character: use the patient's words to note character of pain
    (c)   Location: have the patient explain, then have them point it out
    (d)   Exacerbation or remission: what makes it better or worse and is it constant or does it vary in intensity
    (e)   Positional pain: does the pain vary with the change of the patient's position.

24

(f)   Medications/allergies: note any medications whether over the counter or not. Do the medications relate to the problem? Take note of the patient's allergies. **Do not rely on the patient's health record or SF 600.**

(g)   Pertinent facts: facts that lead you to your diagnosis. Usually consist of classical signs and/or symptoms.

(3)   Another method to take a medical history is by using the key phrase "SAMPLE PQRST"

S: Symptoms
A: Allergies
M: Medicine taken
P: Past history of similar events
L: Last meal
E: Events leading up to illness or injury
P: Provocation/Position - what brought symptoms on, where is pain located
Q: Quality - sharp, dull, crushing etc.
R: Radiation - does pain travel
S: Severity/Symptoms Associated with - on scale of 1 to 10, what other symptoms occur
T: Timing/Triggers - occasional, constant, intermittent, only when I do this (Activities, food)

(4)   Past History (PH)
(a)   Other significant illnesses
(b)   Prior admissions
(c)   History of major trauma
(d)   Surgery
(e)   Childhood illnesses
(f)   Neurological history

(5)   Family History
(a)   This is the pertinent history of diseases of the family within the patient's bloodline.
(b)   Any disease traced through the family is important. If no history found, note it on SF600

(6)   Social History (SH)
(a)   Drugs, recreational
(b)   ETOH
(c)   Tobacco
(d)   Over the counter medications

Disposition Plan

Treat illness or injury within prescribed "Ambulatory Patient Care" (HSC PAM 40-7-21) Algorithms

Definition of algorithm
A step by step procedure for solving a problem

Purposes

(1)   Systematic approach to screening patients

(2)   Guidance for minimally trained medical personnel to provide a logical conclusion when dealing with medical problems within the limits of his/her training

Algorithm Dispositions Category

(1)   **PHYSICIAN STAT/Category I** - medical problem (**Emergency**) exist that may be life threatening

      (a)   Requires immediate attention of a physician that can handle circumstance

      (b)   **Notify the physician assistant and the senior medic of a Category I patient if a physician is not present.**

      (a)   First aid should be initiated and ambulance transportation arranged if MTF is outside of hospital

(2)   **PA STAT/Category II** - medical problem may exists that may develop into a life threatening condition if not evaluated on a priority basis by a physician, PA

(3)   **PA TODAY/Category III** - medical condition exists which requires PA evaluation

      (a)   Patient will be screened IAW APC-21 algorithm and then sent to PA

      (b)   Physician or PA will make final disposition

(4)   **SELF-CARE PROTOCOL/Category IV**--condition exists that can be taken care of by individual

      (a)   Instructions and/or medications are offered to individual per algorithm protocol

      (b)   Individual or screener may elect to override self-care protocol and have the patient seen by medical officer

NOTE: Overriding this protocol usually depends on appearance of individual or if medical problem is chronic and self-care has already been attempted without results.

(5)   **HOSPITAL CLINIC REFERRAL/Category V** - medical condition exists that requires evaluation by a specialty clinic (e.g. podiatry, OB/GYN, allergy)

      (a)   Medical officer at MTF must make referral

      (b)   PA may want to attempt treatment care plan at MTF level if qualified personnel and resources are available

Steps in screening patient complaint

(1)   Locate category of chief complaint in table of contents.

      (a)   Category of complaint, EXAMPLE - **Ear, Nose, and Throat (ENT)** Complaints

      (b)   Complaint, EXAMPLE - **sore Throat**

      (c)   Number and page, EXAMPLE - **A-1, 16**

(2)   Review preceding page of algorithm prior to, during, and after patient screening

      (a)   EXAMPLE - important information on the algorithm

(b)　　EXAMPLE - treatment protocol, for instructions and medications to provide patient after screening has been completed

(3)　Begin with Block 1 of algorithm and follow arrows depending on patient's response

(a)　　EXAMPLE - is there a history of recent throat or neck trauma?

(b)　　EXAMPLE - if NO, (go to block 3)

(c)　　EXAMPLE - can the patient touch chin to chest?

(d)　　EXAMPLE - if NO, (go to block 4)

(e)　　EXAMPLE - is temperature 100 F or higher, or is the patient unable to swallow? (Determine ability to swallow by observing the patient)

(f)　　EXAMPLE - if NO, (Category III)

(4)　If disposition is a Category IV, refer to preceding page for treatment protocol.

(a)　　EXAMPLE - **Block 6**, Can the patient clear both ears?

(b)　　EXAMPLE - if YES, (Category IV, Treatment Protocol A-1 (6)

(c)　　Follow protocol for medication and patient instructions

(5)　If disposition is an associated complaint, refer to complaint algorithm and begin at block 1 with new complaint.

(a)　　EXAMPLE - **Block 6**, Can the patient clear both ears?

(b)　　EXAMPLE - if NO, (Screen for Ear Pain, Discomfort, or Drainage, A-2).

(6)　Refer to PA Today, Category III disposition if:

(a)　　Complaint not on list

(b)　　Patient has already tried the treatment protocol without relief

(c)　　Patient will not accept treatment protocol

Information needed in the DD Form 689

(1)　MTF personnel are responsible for making sure DD Form 689 blocks 1 through 9 are correctly filled out by a soldier prior to being evaluated by a screener

(2)　MTF personnel may fill out a sick slip for a soldier if he is unable to due injury, illness, or reporting directly to the MTF in the event of an emergency

(3)　All military forms will be filled out in black ink

(4)　**Block 1** - box checked by individual that best fits remarks section (block 8)

(a)　Illness--acute or chronic, (e.g. common cold symptoms, athletes foot, nausea, vomiting, etc.)

(b)　Injury--acute (e.g. direct/indirect trauma within 24 to 48 hours)

(5)　**Block 2** - date

(6)　**Block 3** - name (e.g. complete last, first, middle initial, Doe, Johnny E.)

(7)　**Block 4** - service number. SSN (e.g. complete 9 digits, 000-11-0000)

(8)　**Block 5** - grade/rank (e.g. pay grade, E-1, etc.)

(9)   **Block 6** - organization and Station (e.g. C Co. 232D Medical
        Battalion, Ft. Sam Houston, TX 78234)
(10)   **Block 7** - in line of duty (e.g. yes/no depending on circumstances)
        (a)   Company or unit commander ONLY fills out this block
                when injury occurs
        (b)   Often left blank unless negligence is suspected (e.g.
                soldier was intoxicated at time of injury, or was not at
                his/her appointed place of duty at time of injury etc.)
(11)   **Block 8** - remarks (e.g. sore throat and cough x4 days; right ankle
        pain, difficulty walking due to injury x24 hrs.)
        (a)   Filled out by individual
        (b)   Includes chief complaint (c/o). (e.g. sore throat; right ankle
                pain)
        (c)   Associated illnesses/pain. (e.g. cough; difficulty walking)(d)
                        How long? problem(s) have existed or when
                injury occurred. (e.g. x4 days; x24 Hrs)
(12)   **Block 9** - signature of unit commander.
        (a)   First line supervisor or person who is in charge of quarters
                (CQ) may sign for unit commander (per unit SOP)
        (b)   Individual signing the sick call slip must be in individual's
                immediate chain of command
(13)   **Block 10** - in line of duty (e.g. yes/no or left blank).
(14)   **Block 11** - disposition of patient.
(15)   **Block 12** - remarks (e.g. Quarters x24 Hrs, return in A.M. for follow
        up or Profiling e.g. no running or marching x5 days)
        (a)   Remarks reflect box checked in block 11
        (b)   Also indicates:
                (i)   Soldier's arrival time at MTF
                (ii)   Soldier's disposition
                (iii)   Time of release back to unit

(16)   **Block 13**--signature of medical officer **ONLY**
(17)   Disposition of DD Form 689
        (a)   DD Form 689 is returned to individual after medical
                evaluation has been completed
        (b)   Soldier returns original sick slip to first line supervisor or
                per unit SOP
        (c)   Soldier keeps copy of sick slip if quarters or profile given

TERMINAL LEARNING OBJECTIVE

Given an order to deploy, ensure proper immunization and chemoprophylaxis IAW AR 40-562.

Personnel subject to immunizations and required shots

All active duty personnel are subject to immunizations

Specific Requirements

(1)   Anthrax - not being administered at present
    (a)   Dosage Schedule
        (i)   Full immunity requires six doses administered at 0, 2, and 4 weeks, and at 6, 12, and 18 months, to complete the primary series. This schedule is the only schedule approved by the FDA at this time. Annual boosters are required.
        (ii)   Doses of the vaccine should not be administered on a compressed or accelerated schedule (for example, shorter intervals between doses or more doses than required).
    (b)   Medical exemptions can only be granted by a medical officer (MD/PA)
    (c)   Adverse Events
        (i)   Localized injection site reactions-redness, pain
        (ii)   Serious adverse reactions are rare
(2)   Cholera
    (a)   Cholera vaccine is not administered routinely
    (b)   Only administered to military personnel, upon travel or deployment to countries requiring cholera vaccination as a condition for entry
    (c)   Adverse Events:
        (i)   Pain at injection site, mild systemic complaints, and temperature > 37.7 C
        (ii)   Local reaction may be accompanied by fever, malaise, and headache
        (iii)   Serious reactions, including neurologic reactions, after cholera vaccination are extremely rare
(3)   Hepatitis A
    (a)   Use Hepatitis A vaccine and immune globulin (IG) according to Army Command Immunization Program (ACIP) and Service - specific guidance
    (b)   Adverse events: Rare
(4)   Hepatitis B
    (a)   Given to health care workers and soldiers PCSing to Korea.

        (b)   Adverse Events: Pain at injection site, mild systemic complaints, and temperature > 37.7 C

(5)   Influenza

        (a)   All active duty and reserve military personnel entering active duty for periods in excess of 30 days are immunized against influenza soon after entry on active duty

        (b)   The vaccine is provided to all health care providers and others considered to be at high risk for influenza infection

        (c)   Adverse Events: Local reactions, fever/malaise (common) severe allergic reactions, and neurological reactions (rare)

(6)   Japanese B Encephalitis (JE)

        (a)   Specific guidance on indication for use and schedule of immunization in military populations is provided by the each service

        (b)   Adverse Events: Fever, headache, myalgias, malaise (common). General urticaria, angioedema, respiratory distress, and anaphylaxis (rare).

(7)   Measles, Mumps, and Rubella (MMR)

        (a)   Measles and rubella are administered to all recruits regardless of prior history

        (b)   Mumps or MMR vaccine is administered to persons considered to be mumps susceptible. Written documentation of physician diagnosed mumps or a documented history of prior receipt of live virus mumps vaccine or MMR vaccine is adequate evidence of immunity.

        (c)   Adverse Events: Low grade fever, parotitis, rash, pruritis (mild), deafness (rare)

(8)   Meningococcus

        (a)   Meningococcal vaccine is administered on a one-time basis to recruits.

        (b)   Adverse Events-rare

(9)   Plague

        (a)   There are no requirements for routine immunization. Plague vaccine is administered to soldiers who are likely to be assigned to areas where the risk of endemic transmission or other exposure is high.

        (b)   The addition of antibiotic prophylaxis is recommended for such situations.

        (c)   Adverse Events: General malaise, headache, fever, mild lymphadenopathy, and/or erythema, and induration at the injection site

(10)   Polio

        (a)   A single dose of trivalent OPV is administered to all enlisted recruits. Officer candidates, ROTC cadets, and other Reserve Components on initial active duty for training receive a single dose of OPV unless prior booster immunization as an adult is documented.

        (c)   Booster doses of OPV are not routinely administered

        (d)   Adverse Events

    (i) Paralytic poliomyelitis: more likely in immunodeficient persons, no procedure available for identifying persons at risk of paralytic disease (rare).

(11) Rabies

  (a) Preexposure Series. Rabies vaccine is administered to personnel with a high risk of exposure (animal handlers; certain laboratory, field, and security personnel; and personnel frequently exposed to potentially rabid animals in a nonoccupational or recreational setting).

  (b) Post exposure Series. Rabies vaccine and rabies immune globulin (RIG) administration will be coordinated with appropriate medical authorities following current ACIP recommendations.

  (c) Adverse Events: Anaphylaxis (rare)

(12) Smallpox

  (a) This vaccine is administered only under the authority of the Immunization Program for Biological Warfare Defense

  (b) Adverse events: Person can become infected with the smallpox virus.

(13) Tetanus-Diphtheria

  (a) A primary series of tetanus-diphtheria (Td) toxoid is initiated for all recruits lacking a reliable history of prior immunization. Individuals with previous history of Td immunization receive a booster dose upon entry to active duty and every 5-10 years thereafter.

  (b) Adverse events

    (i) Local reactions (erythema, induration)

    (ii) Nodule at injection site

    (iii) Fever and systemic symptoms uncommon

(14) Typhoid

  (a) Typhoid vaccine is administered to alert forces and personnel deploying to endemic areas. Either oral or intramuscular vaccine is used.

  (b) Adverse Events

    (i) Local reactions maybe accompanied by fever, malaise, and headache (common)

    (ii) Nausea

    (iii) Abdominal cramps

    (iv) Vomiting

    (v) Skin rash

    (vi) Urticaria

(15) Yellow Fever

  (a) Yellow fever immunization is required for all alert forces, active duty personnel or Reserve Components traveling to yellow fever endemic areas.

  (b) Adverse events:

    (i) Mild headache, myalgia, low grade fever, other minor symptoms

(ii)   Immediate hypersensitivity reactions: rash, urticaria, and asthma. Uncommon and occur periodically among people with a history of egg allergies

Chemoprophylactic Requirements

(1)   Command medical officers review indications for use and potential adverse effects of specific chemoprophylactic medications prior to use. Current ACIP(Advisory Committee on Immunization Practices) or Control of Communicable Disease Manual recommendations and consultation with the relevant preventive medicine authority are followed for the use of chemoprophylactic agents for the following diseases which have historically been shown to be of military significance:
   (a)   Influenza
   (b)   Meningococcal disease
   (c)   Leptospirosis
   (d)   Plague
   (e)   Scrub typhus
   (f)   Traveler's diarrhea

Malaria

(1)   Comprehensive malaria prevention counseling includes mosquito avoidance and personal protective measures (clothing, repellents, bednetting, etc.). Chemoprophylaxis is provided to military and civilian personnel considered to be at risk of contracting malaria. Specific chemoprophylactic regimens are determined by each of the services based on degree and length of exposure and the prevalence of drug resistance strains of Plasmodia in the area(s) of travel.

Group A Streptococcal Disease

(1)   Each service develops policies for surveillance and prophylaxis of streptococcal disease at recruit centers

Pre-administration Screening

Medical record screening

(1)   What immunizations are required for this individual?
   (a)   Routine immunizations are identified in AR 40-562 and local policy
   (b)   Additional requirements specific for deployment:
      (i)   Based on disease prevalence in specific geographic regions

        (ii)   Determined by Preventive Medicine using Federal, Department of Defense, and other relevant sources of information

(2)   Current immunization status:
    (a)   What has been given?
    (b)   When?
    (c)   Initial series completed?
    (d)   Are boosters current?

(3)   What immunizations are needed, if any, to meet current update/deployment requirements?

(4)   If pre-deployment, is there time to administer all required vaccine series/boosters before date of departure? If not, is an exception to policy needed?

(5)   Does the medical record reflect any contraindications for immunization?

Patient screening

(1)   It is **YOUR** responsibility to ask the patient about allergies, pregnancy, or current illness **BEFORE** administering the vaccine

(2)   Refer patients with any risk factors to the medical officer for disposition

Vaccine Handling, Administrative, and Patient Care Procedures

Vaccine handling

(1)   Pre-immunization
    (a)   Check expiration date/time

    (b)   Evaluate for potential mishandling or contamination
        (i)   Proper storage temperature
            *   Refrigerated vaccines - 35.6 to 46.4^0 F
            *   Frozen vaccines - 0 to 5^0 F or as directed by manufacturer.
        (ii)   Evidence of bacterial growth
        (iii)   Color change/clarity of solution

(2)   Post-immunization
    (i)   Store partially used vials at proper temperature
    (ii)   All live virus vaccine containers should be handled as infectious waste and disposed in biohazard containers to be burned, boiled, or autoclaved, follow local SOP.

Administrative procedures

(1)   Pre-immunization
    (a)   Screen medical record

        (b)   Select correct equipment (needles and syringes) for immunizations to be administered

        (c)   Document vaccine lot number and other identifying information as required by local SOP

(2)   Post-immunization

        (a)   Document all vaccines given in patient medical record (SF 601) IAW local SOP

        (b)   Record immunizations in individual shot record (PHS 731)

        (c)   Record any reactions or side effects

Patient care procedures

(1)   Pre-immunization

        (a)   Ask about contraindications for immunization (allergies, pregnancy, illness etc.)

        (b)   Implement appropriate infection control procedures

        (c)   Explain procedure to patient

        (d)   Position patient and administer required immunizations

(2)   Post-immunization

        (a)   Inform patient when he is to return for next injection in series/booster

        (b)   Instruct patient to wait in facility for observation for 20 minutes (or IAW local SOP)

        (c)   Assure patient is evaluated during and at end of designated waiting period for signs of an adverse reaction

Reactions and possible side effects

Vaccine components can cause allergic reactions in some recipients

Prior to the administration of any immunizing agents, determine if the individual has previously shown any adverse reactions to a specific agent or vaccine component

Vaccine components that can cause reactions include:

(1)   Vaccine antigen (a substance that causes the formation of an antibody)

(2)   Animal proteins

(3)   Antibiotics (e.g., penicillin or penicillin derivatives)

(4)   Preservatives (e.g., thimerosal, a mercurial compound)

(5)   Stabilizers

The most common animal protein allergen is egg protein

Vaccination during pregnancy

(1)   Ideally, all immunizations should precede pregnancy.

(2)   Live virus vaccines are contraindicated (Yellow fever, MMR, OPV)

(3)   Refer pregnant soldiers to medical officer for disposition.
(4)   Breast-feeding - Refer soldier to the medical officer (MD, PA) for disposition

Vaccination with significant illness

(1)   Persons should not be vaccinated if they have moderate or severe febrile illness (usually 101o F or higher, per local SOP)
(2)   Persons should be vaccinated as soon as they recover from the acute phase of the illness
(3)   Minor illnesses, such as diarrhea, mild upper-respiratory infection with or without low-grade fever, or other low-grade febrile illness are not contraindicated to vaccination

HIV positive status – due to compromised immune system, vaccines should not be administered to any patient who has tested positive for HIV, unless specifically ordered by the attending physician with knowledge of the diagnosis

Multiple vaccines

(1)   Contraindicated Combinations/Cautions
          (a)   Do not administer cholera, plague, and/or typhoid vaccines together unless deploying immediately
          (b)   Multiple live virus vaccines may be given the same day. IF THEY ARE NOT GIVEN THE SAME DAY, they must be separated by 30 days. Live virus vaccines are: oral polio, yellow fever, measles, mumps, rubella, and adenovirus.
          (c)   Gamma globulin (immune serum globulin) and MMR must be given at least 14 days apart; if closer together, MMR may be partially or completely ineffective in protecting against disease. If closer administration is unavoidable, MMR must be repeated after three months. Gamma globulin administration does not reduce effectiveness of inactivated vaccines.
          (d)   A PPD TB test and live vaccines may be given the same day. IF NOT GIVEN THE SAME DAY, the TB test must be deferred for 6 weeks after the live vaccine is given, to prevent a false negative result from the TB test.
(2)   No more than one vaccine should be administered in any one anatomical site.

Documentation

DHHS Form PHS 731 is prepared for each member of the Armed Forces and for nonmilitary personnel.

(1)   Valid certificates of immunization for international travel and quarantine purposes.

(2)   Remains in the custody of the individual who is responsible for its safekeeping and for keeping it in his or her possession when performing international travel.

(3)   Entries based on prior official records have the following statement added: "Transcribed from official U.S. Department of Defense records."

(4)   Obtained through normal publication supply channels. The DOD Immunization Stamp is available through medical supply channels.

National vaccine injury compensation program

(1)   Information is recorded on PHS Form 731, medical record and on the clinic log or equivalent computer data base. Information includes, name, sponsor's SSN, date of administration, type of vaccine, manufacturer, lot number, and the name, address, and title of person administering the vaccine.

(2)   In addition, all health care providers who administer any vaccine containing diphtheria, tetanus, pertussis, measles, mumps, rubella, or polio to either children or adults must provide a copy of the most recent relevant vaccine information materials provided by the DHHS

Issuance of DHHS Form PHS 731 to Military Personnel

(1)   At the time of initial immunization of a person entering military services, DHHS Form PH 731 and SF 601, Health Records-Immunization Records, are initiated as outlined below. Written statements from civilian physicians attesting to immunization with approved vaccines, and providing dates and dosages, are accepted as evidence of immunization. Such information is transcribed to official records. Immunizations are recorded on the cited forms, and the forms are maintained as follows.

(2)   Army, Navy, and Marine Corps. SF 601 is prepared in accordance with AR 40-66, Medical Records and Quality Assurance Administration, And Chapter 16, NAVMED P-107, Manual of the Medical Department, U.S. Navy. When prepared, SF 601 and DHHS Form 731 contain the SSN as identifying data

Issuance of DHHS Form PHS 731 to Nonmilitary Personnel

(1)   At the time of initial immunization of nonmilitary personnel, entries are made on DHHS Form PHS 731, which is retained by the individual. All subsequent immunizations are recorded on this form which can be presented as an official record of immunizations received. In addition to DHHS Form PHS 731, SF 601 (Army, Navy and Marine Corps) or SF 600 (Air Force) is prepared and permanently maintained for each individual. Individuals preparing the DHHS Form PHS 731 and SF 601(600) ensure appropriate entries are recorded on both forms and both forms are current and agree with one another.

TERMINAL LEARNING OBJECTIVE

Given the appropriate equipment and guidance, you will be able to collect specimens for diagnostic testing

General principles for throat culture and sputum collection

Throat culture
(1)   A sample of both the mucus and the secretions from the back of the throat is obtained on a cotton tipped applicator and applied to a slide or culture medium, which is then incubated in the laboratory to determine what organism if any is present.

(2)   Drug sensitivity determinations may also be done to determine which drug is most effective against a particular organism. This test also determines which drugs the organism is resistant to.

(3)   A culture may be done within a matter of hours to rule out the presence of the streptococcus organism. This test does not rule out any other organism. The quick strep test is done in cases of suspected strep infection, so that antibiotic therapy can be initiated.

Sputum specimens
(1)   Reasons for cytology study
     (a)   Study cells that may be malignant
     (b)   Determine organisms causing infection
     (c)   Identify blood or pus in the sputum

Collection implications
(1) Sputum is best obtained in the morning, before breakfast, after secretions have accumulated in the respiratory tract during the night

(2)   Usually, specimens are collected on 3 successive days

(3)   Best to have the patient brush their teeth and rinse their mouth so saliva and oral debris do not contaminate the specimen

(4)   Patient should be taught that sputum is matter ejected from the lower respiratory tract through the mouth and that saliva is an unsatisfactory specimen.

(5)   Patient should be instructed to inhale deeply and cough deeply on exhalation. About a teaspoon of sputum is needed for a specimen.

(6)   Sputum should be coughed directly into a sterile specimen container that is then covered with a sterile lid, properly labeled, and sent to the laboratory

(7)   A note should be charted in the patient's record about the character of the sputum, including amount, appearance, and odor

(8)   Explain to patient that if sputum cannot be obtained, an induced sputum specimen may be required

NOTE: Precautions should be taken in the care and disposal of sputum. Gloves and a mask should be worn and hands washed after contact with sputum. All tissues are discarded as contaminated material.

Stool specimens

General principles

(1)   Reason - stool specimen yields information about the patient related to the functioning of the gastrointestinal system and its accessory organs (See C191W026, Treat Gastrointestinal Symptoms)
(2)   Explain the reason for the test to the patient
(3)   The best time of day to collect a stool specimen is soon after breakfast
(4)   Patient should be instructed that a stool specimen is to be saved
(5)   Patient should be instructed to notify the soldier medic as soon as there is an urge to defecate
(6)   Give the bedpan to the patient when they are ready
(7)   Use tongue blades and wear gloves when transferring the stool specimen to the specimen cup
(8)   Some specimens must be kept warm to keep any parasites alive until the specimen is examined in the laboratory
(9)   Always label the specimen container with the patient's name, SSN and all pertinent information
(10)   Always send an appropriate lab slip with the container

Guaiac test

(1)   Purpose - to ascertain the presence of occult blood that is not visible
(2)   Each method of testing has a specific procedure that must be followed in order to obtain accurate results (i.e. food restrictions and number of days to collect smear)
(3)   Manufacturer's instructions or hospital procedure manual should be consulted for specifics

Urine specimens

General principles

(1)   Urinalysis is the laboratory examination of a urine specimen. Analysis of the urine is a common way of securing data about a person's health state.
(2)   The soldier medic is responsible for instructing the patient about urine collection techniques or for obtaining specimen from the patient
(3)   A cooperative patient can be instructed to put specimen into a clean or, in some instances, a sterile container. Care should be taken that the outside of the container is not contaminated.

NOTE: Precautions similar to those when handling blood are appropriate with all body fluids.

Mid-stream (clean-catch)

(1)   Reason for obtaining a mid-stream:

(a) Obtain a sample that has been in the bladder an extended period of time

(b) Provide accurate information of the function of the kidneys the presents of pathogenic organisms, and the excretion of electrolytes that are normally use for normal body functions (i.e., potassium)

(2) Patient voids a little urine, which is discarded; the specimen is collected during mid-stream, and the last urine in the bladder is also discarded

(3) Procedure

   (a) Wear gloves

   (b) For the female

      (i) Spread the labia well, and keep them apart until the specimen is obtained.

      (ii) Clean the area at the external meatus with sterile gauze or cotton balls and antiseptic soap and water.

         * Move the gauze or cotton balls from the meatus toward the anus

         * Use one piece of gauze or one cotton ball for each stroke

      (iii) Have the patient void about 30 cc then discard this urine

      (iv) Position the sterile specimen container near but not touching the meatus and ask them to void forcibly if she is lying down. This prevents collecting a specimen that has dribbled down across the perineal area.

   (c) For the male

      (i) Retract the foreskin to expose the glans penis in the uncircumcised male patient

      (ii) Clean the area of the external meatus with sterile gauze or cotton balls and antiseptic soap and water

         * Move gauze or cotton ball in a circular manner at the meatus, and move down the shaft of the penis a few inches

         * Use one piece of gauze or one cotton ball for each stroke

      (iii) Have the patient void about 30 cc then discard this urine

      (iv) Have patient void directly into the sterile container

      (v) Have patient stop before he empties bladder

      (vi) Return foreskin to its normal position to prevent swelling and irritation of the glans penis

NOTE: With male patients, a sterile urinal may be used if unable to urinate into cup. With female patients, a sterile bedpan may be used if unable to urinate into cup.

(d)   Label specimen container appropriately and send specimen to the laboratory

Blood cultures are used to identify a disease-causing organism especially in patients who spike temperatures for unknown reasons

Procedure

(1)   Explain the reason for the procedure to the patient
(2)   Gather all supplies and equipment and bring to the patient's bedside
(3)   Make the patient as comfortable as possible in bed
(4)   If patient is uncooperative or disoriented you may need assistance
(5)   Clean the tops of all bottles with a betadine solution
(6)   Attach the needle to the syringe
(7)   Apply the tourniquet
(8)   Don gloves and clean the drawing site with a betadine solution
(9)   Wash hands
(10)   Draw at least 10 cc of blood from the patient (5 cc's is needed for each bottle)
(11)   Loosen the tourniquet
(12)   Remove the syringe and needle while applying pressure to the site
(13)   Replace the needle on the syringe with another sterile needle
(14)   Inject 5 cc of blood into anaerobic bottle and do not allow air to enter the bottle
(15)   Replace the needle on the syringe with another sterile needle
(16)   Inject 5 cc of blood in the aerobic bottle and while the needle is still in the bottle, disconnect it from the syringe so that air enters the aerobic bottle, if IAW local SOP.
(17)   Gently mix the blood with the solution in both bottles
(18)   Label both bottles with patient identifying information and type of culture, ie, aerobic or anaerobic
(19)   Prepare lab slip and take slips and specimens to the lab immediately
(20)   Place a band aid over the patient's venipuncture site

TERMINAL LEARNING OBJECTIVE

Obtain a blood specimen while maintaining aseptic technique and without causing injury to the patient.

General Considerations

Terms and definitions
(1)   Venipuncture - the transcutaneous puncture of a vein to withdraw a specimen of blood, start an IV or instill a medication
(2)   Palpate - to feel or to examine by hand
(3)   Antecubital fossa - hollow or depressed area at the bend of the elbow
(4)   Anticoagulant - substance that prevents or delays clotting of the blood
(5)   Hematoma - swelling or mass of blood confined to an organ, tissue, or space and caused by a break in a blood vessel

Veins used for drawing blood
(1)   Median cubital vein - first choice, well supported, least apt to roll
(2)   Cephalic vein - second choice
(3)   Basilic vein - third choice, often the most prominent vein, but it tends to roll easily and makes venipuncture difficult

Steps and Procedures to Perform a Venipuncture

CAUTION: Universal precautions for this task will include hand washing and gloves.

CAUTION: Strict adherence to the sharps policy and the use of sharps containers will be utilized during this hands on exercise.

Verify the request to obtain a blood specimen. Check the physician's orders
Select the proper blood specimen tube for the test to be performed. Check local laboratory SOP
(1)   The type of blood tube needed will depend on the specific test to be performed
      (2)   For some tests, an anticoagulant or other additives are present in the tube
(3)   Rubber stoppers of the tubes are color-coded for different tests
Prepare label(s)
(1)   Stamp label with patient's addressograph plate. If there is no plate, write name, organization, social security number, prefix code, ward or clinic, facility, and date.
(2)   Apply to specimen tube
Perform a patient care hand wash/don gloves
Gather equipment
(1)   Constricting band
(2)   Vacutainer sleeve/holder
(3)   Sterile disposable double-ended needle

(a)   Single specimen vacutainer needle
(b)   Multiple samples - a rubber sheath covers the shaft of the needle. It is pushed up when the blood tube is inserted onto the needle then slips back over the needle holder while tubes are being changed to prevent blood from dripping into holder
(4)   Betadine or alcohol wipe or sponge

CAUTION: Always ask the patient if he/she has an allergy to iodine or Betadine before applying.

(5)   Protective pad (chux)
(6)   Sterile 2 x 2-inch gauze sponge(s)
(7)   Band-Aid
Assemble vacutainer and needle
(1)   Put short end of needle into threaded hole in vacutainer
(2)   Screw tightly using clockwise motion
Insert rubber stoppered end of the specimen tube into vacutainer holder and advance the tube until it is even with the guideline

CAUTION: If the tube is pushed beyond the guideline, the vacuum may released and blood will not be pulled into the tube.

Identify patient

Explain the procedure and purpose for collecting the blood specimen to the patient

CAUTION: Ask patient about allergies (i.e., iodine or alcohol).

Position the patient - sitting or lying

CAUTION: Never attempt to draw blood from a standing patient.

Position protective pad under patient's extended elbow and forearm

Expose area for venipuncture
(1)   Roll garment above the elbow
(2)   Extend patient's arm with palm up
Select vein for venipuncture - Palpate and select one of the most prominent veins in antecubital fossa

CAUTION: You may need to apply the constricting band at this point for venipuncture site selection.

Prepare sponges for use
(1)   Open the betadine or alcohol and 2 x 2 gauze sponge packages
(2)   Place them within easy reach (still in the packages)
Apply constricting band with enough pressure to stop venous return without stopping the arterial flow. A radial pulse should be felt

(1)   Wrap latex tubing around limb about 2 inches above venipuncture
         site
(2)   Stretch tubing slightly and hold with one end longer than the other
(3)   Loop longer end and draw under shorter end so tails are away from
         site
(4)   If a commercial band is used, wrap it around limb as in step 14a and
         secure by overlapping Velcro ends.
(5)   Instruct patient to clench and unclench his fist several times and then
         hold clenched fist to trap blood in veins and distend them.

CAUTION: Avoid veins that are infected, injured, irritated, or have an IV running
                 distally.

Palpate selected vein
(1)   Palpate along length of vein with index finger up and down 1 or 2
         inches from selected site in both directions so size and direction of
         vein can be determined.
(2)   Vein should feel like a spongy tube
**Clean the skin - moving alcohol/betadine wipe in a circular motion away
from selected venipuncture site.**

CAUTION: Do not repalpate the vein after cleansing the skin.

Prepare to puncture vein
(1)   Remove protective cover from needle
(2)   Position needle in line with vein and grasp patient's arm below entry
         point with free hand
(3)   Place thumb of free hand 1 inch below entry site and pull skin taut
         toward hand
Puncture vein
(1)   Align needle, bevel up, with the vein and pierce skin at 15 to 30
         degree angle
(2)   Decrease angle until almost parallel to skin surface, then pierce vein
         wall
         (a)   A faint "give" will be felt when the vein is entered, and
                 blood will appear in the needle
         (b)   If venipuncture is unsuccessful, pull needle back slightly
                 (not above the skin surface), and redirect needle toward
                 vein and try again

CAUTION: If needle is withdrawn above skin surface, do not attempt
                 venipuncture again with the same needle.

         (c)   If still unsuccessful
                 (i)   Release the constricting band
                 (ii)   Place 2 x 2 gauze sponge over site
                 (iii)   Quickly withdraw the needle and instruct the
                         patient to elevate arm slightly and keeping the
                         arm fully extended apply pressure to the site for
                         2 to 3 minutes.

(iv)   Notify supervisor before attempting another venipuncture

Collect the specimen

(1)   Single specimen

    (a)   Hold vacutainer unit and needle steady with dominant hand. Collection tube is positioned against, but not through, the needle

    (b)   Place index and middle fingers of other hand behind flange of vacutainer

    (c)   Push the tube as far forward as possible with thumb of nondominant hand without causing excessive movement

    (d)   Instruct patient to relax and unclench fist after blood has started flowing

    (e)   Release the constricting band by pulling on long end of looped tubing or releasing Velcro fastener with the non dominant hand

    (f)   When tube is about two-thirds full of blood or blood stops, grasp tube firmly and remove tubes

    (g)   Prepare to withdraw needle

(2)   Multiple specimens

    (a)   Follow same steps for collecting single specimen

    (b)   Remove first tube from vacutainer sleeve without dislodging needle position

    (c)   Insert second tube into vacutainer sleeve. Push tube as far forward as possible without causing excessive movement.

    (d)   Repeat these procedures until the desired number of tubes are filled or blood stops flowing

    (e)   Release the constricting band by pulling on long end of looped tubing or releasing Velcro fastener with the non dominant hand.

CAUTION: DO NOT withdraw the needle before the constricting band is released because of potential for heavy blood loss and/or hematoma formation.

    (f)   After the last tube is about two-thirds full of blood or blood stops, grasp tube firmly and remove tubes

    (g)   Place 2 x 2-inch sponge lightly over venipuncture site

    (h)   Withdraw the needle smoothly and quickly. Immediately apply pressure to the site with the 2 x 2-inch sponge, keeping patient's arm fully extended.

    (i)   Instruct the patient to elevate arm slightly and keeping the arm fully extended, apply firm manual pressure for 2 to 3 minutes. If the patient is unable to do this for himself, you must do it for him.

If specimen tube contains an anticoagulant or other additive, gently invert tube several times to mix with blood

Apply a band aid to the venipuncture site after the bleeding has stopped

CAUTION: Dispose of needle into sharps container as soon as possible or IAW local protocol. DO NOT unscrew needle from sleeve with hands. DO NOT recap needle.

Provide for patient's comfort and safety
(1)   Remove protective pad
(2)   Roll down patient's sleeve
(3)   Reposition patient and raise side rails if patient is in a bed

Dispose of equipment
(1)   Remove all the equipment from area
(2)   Dispose of used supplies
(3)   Store reusable equipment and dispose of needle IAW local SOP
(4)   Remove gloves and wash hands

Administrative duties:
(1)   Check and complete laboratory form IAW local SOP
(2)   Apply prepared label(s) to specimen tube(s)
(3)   Document procedure IAW local SOP

Appendix A
Specimen Collection
Competency Skill Sheets

D Stick

Soldiers Name: _____ SSN: _____ CO: _____ TM:
_____

Start: _____ Stop: _____ Initial Evaluator: _____
Start: _____ Stop: _____ Retest Evaluator: _____
Start: _____ Stop: _____ Final Evaluator: _____

		1st	2nd	3rd
a.	Gathers equipment.	P / F	P / F	P / F
b.	Identifies patient and explains procedure to patient.	P / F	P / F	P / F
c.	Performs patient care handwash.	P / F	P / F	P / F
d.	Dons gloves.	P / F	P / F	P / F
e.	Removes cap from lancet using sterile technique.	P / F	P / F	P / F
f.	Selects site on patient's fingertip.	P / F	P / F	P / F
g.	Wipes selected site with alcohol swab.	P / F	P / F	P / F
h.	Asks patient to hold arm at side for 30 seconds.	P / F	P / F	P / F
i.	Gently squeezes patient's fingertip with thumb of same hand.	P / F	P / F	P / F
j.	Hold lancing device and places trigger platform of lancing device on same side of finger and presses.	P / F	P / F	P / F
k.	Squeezes finger in a downward motion, wiping off first drop of blood.	P / F	P / F	P / F
l.	While holding strip level, touch drop of blood to test pad.	P / F	P / F	P / F
m.	Begin recommended timing. After 60 seconds, blot blood off test strip into appropriate site on meter. Wait for numeric readout.	P / F	P / F	P / F
n.	Discards lancet into a sharps container.	P / F	P / F	P / F
o.	Removes gloves and discards.	P / F	P / F	P / F
p.	Documents procedure.	P / F	P / F	P / F

Instructor Comments:

Dip UA

Soldiers Name: _____ SSN: _____ CO: _____ TM: _____
Start: _____ Stop: _____ Initial Evaluator: _____
Start: _____ Stop: _____ Retest Evaluator: _____
Start: _____ Stop: _____ Final Evaluator: _____

		1st	2nd	3rd
a.	Instructs patient to collect a mid-stream catch UA.	P / F	P / F	P / F
b.	Verbalizes that UA testing must be performed within 1 hour of collection.	P / F	P / F	P / F
c.	Dons clean gloves.	P / F	P / F	P / F
d.	Thoroughly mixes specimen and records color and turbidity.	P / F	P / F	P / F
e.	Removes 1 UA strip from bottle and replaces cap.	P / F	P / F	P / F
f.	Completely immerses reagent areas of the strip and removes immediately. While removing, runs the edge of the strip against the rim of the urine container to remove excess urine.	P / F	P / F	P / F
g.	Holds the strip in a horizontal position to prevent mixing of chemicals from adjacent reagent areas.	P / F	P / F	P / F
h.	Compares test areas to corresponding color chart on the bottle label at the times specified. Holds strip close to color blocks and matches carefully.	P / F	P / F	P / F
i.	Documents results.	P / F	P / F	P / F

Instructor Comments:

Clean Catch UA

Soldiers Name: _____ SSN: _____ CO: _____ TM: _____

Start: _____ Stop: _____ Initial Evaluator: _____

Start: _____ Stop: _____ Retest Evaluator: _____

Start: _____ Stop: _____ Final Evaluator: _____

		1st	2nd	3rd
a.	Collects supplies.	P / F	P / F	P / F
b.	Identifies patient.	P / F	P / F	P / F
c.	Explains procedure to patient and ensures that the patient understands how to perform the procedure if patient is able to perform him/herself.	P / F	P / F	P / F
d.	If patient is unable to perform procedure by him/herself: (1) Washes hands and dons clean gloves. (2) Cleans perineum from anterior to posterior with antiseptic solution. Separation the labia on a female patient. Retracts foreskin on an uncircumcised male. Uses each cotton ball saturated with antiseptic solution one time only. (3) Request that patient void about 20ml, then places the sterile specimen container so that the sides of the labia of the female do not touch. Without stopping the flow, have the patient void a small amount into the specimen cup and then finish voiding into the toilet. (4) Secures lid on container (5) Cleans and returns seat collection, if applicable	P / F	P / F	P / F
e.	Labels specimen.	P / F	P / F	P / F
f.	Documents procedure.	P / F	P / F	P / F

Instructor Comments:

Appendix B
Blood Culture
Competency Skill Sheets

Culture

Soldiers Name: _____ SSN: _____ CO: _____ TM: _____

Start: _____ Stop: _____ Initial Evaluator: _____
Start: _____ Stop: _____ Retest Evaluator: _____
Start: _____ Stop: _____ Final Evaluator: _____

		1st	2nd	3rd
a.	Identifies patient and explains the procedure to the patient. Identifies any patient allergies to betadine or medications.	P / F	P / F	P / F
b.	Gathers equipment.	P / F	P / F	P / F
c.	Performs a patient care handwash.	P / F	P / F	P / F
d.	Cleans the tops of all bottles with a betadine solution.	P / F	P / F	P / F
e.	Dons clean gloves.	P / F	P / F	P / F
f.	Attaches needle to the syringe.	P / F	P / F	P / F
g.	Applies tourniquet to patient's arm and cleans site with a betadine solution.	P / F	P / F	P / F
h.	Draws at least 10cc from patient (5cc for each bottle).	P / F	P / F	P / F
i.	Loosens tourniquet and removes syringe and needle while applying pressure to the site.	P / F	P / F	P / F
j.	Replaces the needle on the syringe with another sterile needle without contaminating the equipment or sticking him/herself.	P / F	P / F	P / F
k.	Injects 5 cc of blood into the anaerobic bottle and does not allow air to enter the bottle.	P / F	P / F	P / F
l.	Replaces the needle on the syringe with another sterile needle without contaminating the equipment or sticking him/herself.	P / F	P / F	P / F
m.	Injects 5cc of blood into the aerobic bottle and while the needle is still in the bottle, disconnects it from the syringe so that air enters the aerobic bottle.	P / F	P / F	P / F
n.	Gently mixes the blood with the solution in both bottles.	P / F	P / F	P / F
o.	Removes gloves and discards.	P / F	P / F	P / F
p.	Labels both bottles with patient information and type of culture.	P / F	P / F	P / F
q.	Documents procedure.	P / F	P / F	P / F

Instructor Comments:

This page intentionally left blank.

Clinical Handbook

Supportive Care 3

This page intentionally left blank.

91W10
Advanced Individual
Training Course

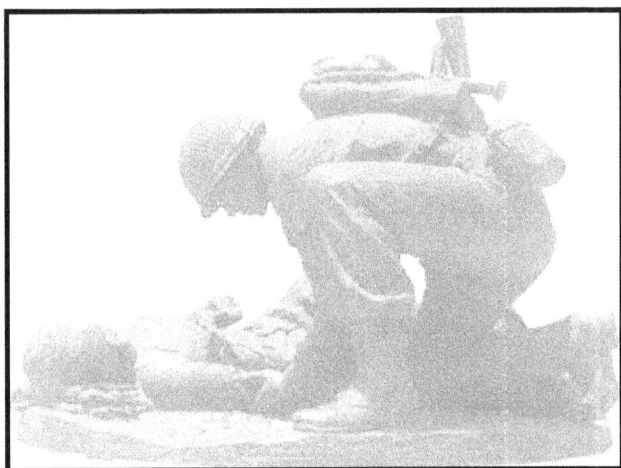

Clinical Handbook
Supportive Care 3

Department of the Army
Academy of Health Sciences
Fort Sam Houston, Texas 78234

TERMINAL LEARNING OBJECTIVE

Given the necessary medical equipment in a holding or ward setting. You are providing casualty care as part of an integrated team in a Minimal Care Ward.

Facts about Physical Assessment

The systematic collection and analysis of subjective and objective data (facts). This information is collected to provide a database.
(1)   Subjective data
(2)   Objective data
(3)   Data Base
Assessment is used to establish a database for the patient. It is the basis on which patient strengths and health problems are identified.

The primary source of patient information is the patient.
Other resources include:
(1)   Patient's support persons
(2)   Patient record
(3)   Information from other health care professionals
The physical assessment is focused primarily on the functional abilities of the patient

Purposes of a physical assessment:

(1)   To confirm the patient's history or to observe findings not reported in the history
(2)   To obtain a physical and mental database on the patient which can be used for nursing intervention
(3)   To evaluate or measure the quality of the care (intervention) given to the patient
Considerations in patient preparation for a physical assessment
(1)   Evaluate all sources of data
        (a)   Patient
        (b)   Support people
        (c)   Patient record
        (d)   Other health professionals
(2)   Exam should occur in a quiet, well-lit room with consideration for patient privacy and comfort
(3)   Explain all procedures to patient to avoid alarming or worrying patient and encourage cooperation
(4)   Ask patient to empty bladder prior to exam and assist with gowning/draping as needed
(5)   Discuss confidentiality with patient

Basic techniques used in performing an assessment

The nursing assessment includes two steps:
(1) Collection and verification of data from a primary source (the patient) and   secondary source (the family, health care professionals)
(2) The analysis of that data to establish a baseline

Inspection: Observations using visual, auditory, and olfactory senses

Palpation: Technique using the sense of touch to gather information about   temperature, turgor, texture, moisture, vibrations, and shape

Auscultation: The act of listening to sound produced within the body with a stethoscope

Percussion: The act of striking one object against another for the purpose   of producing sound (tympany, resonance, hyperresonance, dullness, flatness)

Components of the patient assessment

The interview includes:
(1) Chief Complaint
(2) History of Present Illness
(3) Past Health History
(4) Family Health History
(5) Psychosocial History:
    (a) Age
    (b) Sex/Race
    (c) Marital status
    (d) Number of children
    (e) Occupation
    (f) Education
    (g) Religious affiliation
    (h) Living accommodations

General appearance and behavior assessment.
Items to inspect:
(1) Body build (measure height and weight)
(2) Posture
(3) Gait - coordination of movements and pattern of gait.
(4) Hygiene, grooming - note cleanliness, body odors, appropriate dress for age and environment
(5) Signs of illness - note posture, skin color, respirations, nonverbal communications of pain or distress
(6) Affect, attitude, mood - note speech, facial expressions, ability to relax, eye contact, behavior
(7) Cognitive process - note speech content and patterns, appropriate verbal responses

(8)   Cognitive function - an intellectual process by which one becomes aware of, perceives, or comprehends ideas. It involves all aspects of perception, thinking, reasoning, and remembering.

Vital Signs

(1)   Temperature:
- (a)   May vary with the time of day
- (b)   Oral: 98.6 degrees Fahrenheit is considered normal
- (c)   Rectal temperature is most accurate. Temperature of > 100.4 = fever.

(2)   Blood Pressure
- (a)   Measure the blood pressure in both arms
- (b)   Use the correct sized cuff
  - (i)   To determine cuff size, the length of the cuff should be 80% of the upper arm circumference and be two-thirds the width of the upper arm.
  - (ii)   An improper size will give an inaccurate reading. A higher inaccurate reading will be obtained if too small a cuff is used. conversely, a lower inaccurate reading will be obtained if too large a cuff is used.
- (c)   Normal range 95-140 mmHg systolic, 60-90 mmHg diastolic

(3)   Pulse
- (a)   Palpate pulses for at least 30 seconds
- (b)   Normal adult pulse 60-80 beats/minute
- (c)   Note the number of irregular beats per minute
- (d)   Peripheral pulses are graded on a scale of 0-4 by the following system
  - (i)   0 = Absent, no pulse
  - (ii)   +1 = Not easily felt, thready, weak
  - (iii)   +2 = Difficult to palpate, stronger than +1
  - (iv)   +3 = Normal. Easily felt, not easily obliterated with pressure
  - (v)   +4 = Strong, bounding, unable to obliterate with moderate pressure

(4)   Respiration
- (a)   Count number of respirations taken in 15 seconds and multiply by 4
- (b)   Normally 12-20 resp/min

(5)   Measure pulse oxygen saturation (See LP C191W059, Cardiac Monitoring)

Head-To-Toe Assessment

(1)   Integumentary System
- (a)   Ask if patient has been exposed to harmful environmental materials or increased sun exposure, has recent skin changes, or is currently taking   medications
- (b)   Normal skin color
  - (i)   Varies among races and individuals

        (ii)   Ranges from pinkish white to various shades of brown

        (iii)   Exposed areas may vary in color with unexposed areas

        (iv)   Healthy dark skin has a reddish undertone; buccal mucosa, tongue, lips, nails, normally appear pink

(c)   Skin color assessment:

        (i)   Cyanosis - dusky bluish color
              *   Inspect ears, lips, inside of mouth, hands, nailbeds
              *   Caused by respiratory or cardiac diseases, or cold environment (decreased oxygenation)

        (ii)   Jaundice - yellowish color
              *   Inspect skin, mucous membranes, sclera
              *   Caused by liver disease (increased bilirubin)

        (iii)   Pallor - paleness
              *   Inspect face, lips, conjunctival, mucous membranes
              *   Caused by anemia (decreased hemoglobin) or inadequate blood circulation

        (iv)   Erythema - redness
              *   Inspect facial area, localized areas
              *   Caused by blushing, alcohol intake, fever, injury, infection

(d)   Vascularity - bleeding or bruising

        (i)   Ecchymosis - collection of blood in subcutaneous tissues causing purple discoloration

        (ii)   Petechiae - small hemorrhagic spots caused by capillary bleeding

(e)   Lesions - note presence of wounds, scars, rash, etc.

(f)   Note skin temperature and moisture - normally warm and dry

(g)   Skin turgor - fullness or elasticity of skin

(h)   Edema - excess fluid in tissues characterized by swelling with shiny skin

(i)   Edema scale
        0 = None
        +1 = Trace
        +2 = Moderate
        +3 = Deep
        +4 = Very deep

(2)   HEENT - Head, eyes, ears, nose, throat (inspection and palpation)

(a)   Head - size, shape, symmetry, tenderness

(b)   Eyes

4

              (i)   Symmetry, alignment and movement of eyes, eyelashes, eyebrows, eyelids, pupils

              (ii)   Visual acuity and peripheral vision

              (iii)   Pupils are normally black, equal in size, round, smooth

    (c)   Ears

              (i)   Hearing; shape, size, symmetry of external ear

              (ii)   Palpate external ear for pain, edema, lesions

              (iii)   Ear canal should be smooth and pinkish - examine for wax, discharge, foreign bodies

    (d)   Nose/sinuses

              (i)   Assess for nasal patency by occluding one nostril at a time

              (ii)   Examine mucous membranes for color, presence of exudate, growths

              (iii)   Inspect nasal septum for intactness, deviation

              (iv)   Palpate frontal and maxillary sinuses for pain, edema

    (e)   Throat - inspect lips, gums, teeth, tongue, hard and soft palates

              (i)   Uvula normally centered and freely movable

              (ii)   Tonsils normally small, pink, symmetrical in size

(3)   Nervous System / Neurological Assessment

    (a)   Mental Status

              (i)   Orientation level - person, place, time

              (ii)   Observe patients' appearance, general behavior, response to questions, ability to speak clearly

              (iii)   Note memory recall - short and long term

    (b)   Pupillary reaction to light, accommodation, convergence

    (c)   Motor ability - note abnormal balance, gait, or coordination

    (d)   Sensory function - response to pain, light touch

(4)   Thorax and Lungs (Respiratory)

    (a)   Inspection

              (i)   Shape of chest

               (ii)   Breathing patterns

               (iii)   Rate of respirations

                    *   Bradypnea: Rate less than 12 respirations per minute

                    *   Tachypnea: Rate greater than 20 respirations per minute

                    *   Dyspnea: Breathlessness or difficult breathing

                    *   Orthopnea: Shortness of breath when lying down

                    *   Kussmaul: Faster and deeper respirations than normal without pauses

                    *   Cheyne-Stokes: Cyclic pattern which progresses from slow and shallow to fast and deep with a gradual return to

slow and shallow respirations,
followed by a period of apnea
(b)   Palpation - detect areas of sensitivity, chest expansion
during respiration
(c)   Auscultation - auscultate anterior and posterior fields
(upper, middle, and lower lobes)
    (i)   Rales (crackles): fizzing sound produced by
moisture in airways
    (ii)   Rhonchi: Coarse, gurgling sound in bronchial
tubes - low pitched - resulting from air flow
across passages which are narrowed by fluids,
tumors, swelling
    (iii)   Wheezes: Type of rhonchi - squeaky sound -
high pitched
    (iv)   Cough: Note whether the cough is productive or
non-productive and character of secretions
(5)   Cardiovascular System
    (a)   Inspect the neck and epigastric areas for visible pulsations
    (b)   Palpate
        (i)   Pulses
        (ii)   Edema
        (iii)   Capillary refill:
        *   Acceptable - < 3 seconds
        *   Abnormal or sluggish - > 3 seconds
    (c)   Auscultate - Heart sounds
        (a)   Rate - per minute
        (b)   Rhythm - regular or irregular
(6)   Gastrointestinal

NOTE: Be sure the patient has an empty bladder and that he/she is lying flat
with knees slightly flexed.

    (a)   Inspect the general contour of abdomen
        (i)   Flat
        (ii)   Protuberant
        (iii)   Concave
        (iv)   Note local bulges/scars, note color of scars
    (b)   Auscultate

NOTE: This is done before palpation because the latter may alter the
character of bowel sounds.

        (i)   Note character of bowel sounds (clicks and
gurgles produced by movement of air and flatus
in GI tract)
        *   Auscultate each of four quadrants in a
clockwise systematic manner
        *   Normal frequency ranges from 5-34
bowel sounds per minute, described

as audible, hyperactive, hypoactive, or inaudible

NOTE: Listen for 5 minutes in order to distinguish inaudible from audible bowel sounds.

    (c)   Palpate all four quadrants and note:
        (i)   Muscular resistance
        (ii)   Tenderness
        (iii)   Enlargement of organs
        (iv)   Masses

NOTE: Appetite, usual elimination patterns, character of stool, recent changes, artificial orifices, and use of laxatives should be assessed during the interview.

(7)   Genitourinary
    (a)   History of urinary elimination
        (i)   Unusual patterns of elimination
        (ii)   Recent changes
        (iii)   Aids to elimination
        (iv)   Present or past voiding difficulties
    (b)   Inspection
        (i)   Urine
                *   Color
                *   Clarity
                *   Odor
        (ii)   Urethral orifice for signs of inflammation/discharge
        (iii)   Always inspect testis if patient presents with abdomen pain or urinary tract symptoms
    (c)   Palpate suprapubic areas and note:
        (i)   Tenderness
        (ii)   Distension

(8)   Musculoskeletal
    (a)   Inspection and palpation
        (i)   Gait
        (ii)   Muscles
                *   Bilateral symmetry
                *   Tenderness
                *   Strength/tone
        (iii)   Joints
                *   Note active/passive range of motion (ROM) - Joint movements include flexion, extension, hyperextension, abduction, adduction, pronation, supination.
                *   Palpate joints and note - Pain, swelling, nodules, crepitation (grating sound heard on movement)

(iv)   Bones
    *   Note normal contour or prominences,
            symmetry
    *   Document pain, enlargement, and
            changes in contour

Guidelines for documentation of physical assessment

Each body system is assessed for normal and abnormal findings, and documentation should occur in an organized manner
Data should be recorded legibly using correct grammar
Use only standard approved medical abbreviations
Subjective data should be recorded using patient's own words
Do not record data using nonspecific terms, i.e. adequate, good, normal, poor, large - be specific

Nursing Documentation

TERMINAL LEARNING OBJECTIVE
Using approved forms, accurately document patient status, vital signs and care rendered using the SOAPE format.

Purposes
(1)   Primary - Insures that AMEDD personnel have a concise and complete medical history of active-duty personnel
(2)   Assists AMEDD officers in advising commanders on personnel use and retention
(3)   Appraises Army-wide physical fitness and readiness
(4)   Communication - a means of communicating and sharing information on the patient's status throughout the hospitalization with health care team members
(5)   Legal documentation - a legal document and admissible in court as evidence
(6)   Patient care planning - each professional working with the client has access to the client's baseline and ongoing data. Client responds to the treatment plan from day-to-day is documented. Modifications of the plan of care are then based on this data.
(7)   Audit - patient records may be reviewed to evaluate the quality of care received and to improve the quality of care as indicated
(8)   Research - patient records may be studied by researchers to learn how best to recognize or treat health problems
(9)   Education - clinical manifestations of particular health problems, effective treatment methods, and factors affecting client goal achievement are documented
(10)   Historic document - past information may be pertinent concerning a patient's healthcare
(11)   Reimbursement record - insurance companies, Medicare, and Medicaid require written record of treatments, equipment, and diagnostic procedures before they pay the agency
(12)   Decision - analysis-information from the medical record review can be used to provide information for strategic planners to identify needs and/or resources

Confidentiality of medical information
(1)   Medical confidentiality of all patients will be protected as fully as possible.
(2)   Medical information used for disease
        (a)   Diagnosis
        (b)   Treatment
        (c)   Prevention
(3)   Access given to
        (a)   The patient
        (b)   Patient care personnel
        (c)   Medical researchers
        (d)   Medical educators

(4)   Personnel not involved in a patient's care or in medical research will
        not have access to patient information unless the following situations
        apply -
        (a)   Access required by law (court order)
        (b)   Access needed for hospital accreditation
        (c)   Access authorized by patient
(5)   Disclosure of medical information
        (a)   All requests done in writing except in emergency situations
        (b)   Handled by patient administrator
        (c)   Not provided by the 91W

Medical Record Documentation Procedures

Required procedures for making entries

(1)   Legibly typed or handwritten
(2)   In black or blue black ink
(3)   Signed by the individual who made the entry
        (a)   Military personnel - Sign with full payroll signature, rank,
                MOS, branch of service
        (b)   Civilians - Sign with full payroll signature, title, GS
                (paygrade)
(4)   Date in day-month-year sequence
(5)   Capitalized at the beginning
(6)   Written with present or past tense verbs
(7)   Recorded ASAP
(8)   Abbreviated IAW AR 40-60
(9)   Must be clear, concise, and objective
(10)   Include patient identification on patient identification block. Use
        addressograph or write information legibly.
        (a)   Name
        (b)   Rank
        (c)   Social security number
        (d)   Ward/clinic
        (e)   Admission date/date of visit
        (f)   Hospital register number (in patient's only)

Correction procedures for an entry error

(1)   DO -
        (a)   Draw a single line through information
        (b)   Write "Error," the date, and your initials above entry or
                follow local SOP
(2)   DO NOT -
        (a)   Erase or use correction fluid
        (b)   Skip lines
        (c)   Write between lines
        (d)   Chart for someone else
        (e)   Leave blank lines above signature

Content of Medical Record Entries

Done by direct patient care providers

Nursing Entries on the Patient Record

(1)   Concise, comprehensive nursing assessment
(2)   Up-to-date care plan individualized to the client
(3)   Nursing notes
(4)   Flow sheets
(5)   Graphic sheets
(6)   Medication records
(7)   Intake and output record
(8)   Physician and nursing discharge summary
(9)   Other components of patient record include admission sheet, patient history, physician's orders and progress notes, consultations, and laboratory and x-ray reports

Types of Nursing Documentation (Chart)

(1)   Source-oriented record
      (a)   Separate form for each group of health care (e.g., nursing, medical, laboratory, x-ray department)
      (b)   Chronological notes are kept on each form
      (c)   Easy to find record and continue CHARTING
      (d)   Record of care is fragmented and difficult to trace overall care
      (e)   If the Kardex-Care plan is not retained, the care plan must be duplicated in a narrative format

(2)   Focus charting
      (a)   Patient-centered approach to organizing the narrative portion of the medical record
      (b)   Column format to separate topic words or "focus" statements from the body of the note
      (c)   Enhances communication among health team members
      (d)   Quality improvement auditing more efficient

(3)   Charting by exception is a short hand documentation method
      (a)   Must have well-defined standards of practice;
      (b)   Only significant findings and „exceptions" are documented n narrative notes
      (c)   Requires well-established guidelines and clinical experience to identify exceptions
      (d)   Advantages: Decreased charting time, greater emphasis on pertinent data, standardized assessment, and enhanced communication within the healthcare team

(4)   Flow sheets are used with almost all charting formats for documentation of routine care and repeated monitoring
      (a)   Recognized as a useful tool for efficiency
      (b)   Data retrieval easier for quality improvement monitoring

		(c)	Pertinent items from the flow sheet are summarized into the patient care record
		(d)	Duplicate charting is discouraged
	(5)	Computer charting	
		(a)	Computer capacities are in operation for the admission assessment tool
		(b)	Key client data is automatically recorded
		(c)	Adds to the client data base as new data are identified and modifies the plan of care accordingly
		(d)	Receives a work list indicating the treatment, procedures, and medications necessary for the client throughout the shift
		(e)	Documents care immediately using the computer terminal at the client's bedside
	(6)	Problem-Oriented Medical Record (POMR) emphasizes the patient and his or her health problems	
		(a)	All health professionals record on the same forms
		(b)	Interdisciplinary team works together in identifying a master list of client problems
		(c)	Logical way in which to organize information
		(d)	A "problem" is a condition that requires further observation, diagnosis, assessment, and intervention
		(e)	A care plan is developed, based on the identified problem

SOAP/SOAPIE Documentation

(1) S: Subjective Data
   (a) What the patient tells you about his problem
   (b) Usually expressed in the patient's own words. For example, "My throat hurts", or "I am in pain from my broken leg." Patient may have many complaints.
   (c) Important to record exactly what the patient states is the problem

(2) O: Objective Data
   (a) Observations made by the 91W that support or are related to the subjective data
   (b) Record what you observe about the patient. For example, the patient in pain may speak with a loud, agitated voice, or his facial expressions (grimace) might indicate pain. He may be guarding the painful area. Or he may be very quiet and not moving much which would aggravate the pain. Vital signs may indicate increased pain such as pulse is elevated or blood pressure is elevated.
   (c) Important to record all observations made of the patient to include any physical findings

(3) A: Assessment
   (a) This is your interpretation of the patient's problem/condition
   (b) Subjective and objective data is carefully analyzed to reach conclusions regarding the patient's complaint or problem

(4)   P: Plan
- (a)   The plan for dealing with the problem/compliant or situation is recorded here
- (b)   This may include comfort measures, pharmacological interventions, notifying the physician, patient education, etc.
- (c)   Your plan should be concise and should reflect all the information gathered to this point

(5)   Some documentation formats include the I (Intervention) and E (Evaluation) in addition to the SOAP acronym

(6)   I: Intervention
- (a)   This is your plan of action carried out as described
- (b)   For example, patient was medicated with 50 mg of Demerol for his complaint of leg pain rated as 10/10
- (c)   Be sure to record all interventions

(7)   E: Evaluation
- (a)   This is a record of the effectiveness of your plan and intervention
- (b)   For example, patient states that his leg pain is now rated 5/10 30 minutes after receiving the Demerol
- (c)   Important to record patient's response to the intervention whether the intervention was successful or not
- (d)   Unsuccessful intervention requires re-assessment of the problem.

(8)   Documentation should be concise, factual, organized and contain pertinent information

Record special procedures (diagnostics, therapeutic, nursing)
(1)   Time
(2)   Name of procedure
(3)   Person performing procedure
(4)   Instruction to patient
(5)   Description of what was done
(6)   Lab, x-ray reports
(7)   Patient's condition before, during and after procedure. This is extremely important.

Record all medications and/or treatments
(1)   Record vital signs (TPR/BP) before and after all treatments
(2)   Record all medications and/or treatments with responses

Record discharge note
(1)   Date
(2)   Time
(3)   Manner (ambulatory, wheelchair, stretcher)
(4)   Accompanied (parents, ward personnel)
(5)   Medications and/or treatments with schedules
(6)   Discharge information instructions
(7)   Statement that address patient's understanding of discharge plan
(8)   Follow-up visits

End of Shift Reporting
(1)   Means of communication between the outgoing and incoming staff of each shift
(2)   A change of shift report if given by a primary RN or caregiver to the primary RN or caregiver replacing him or her
(3)   May be given in written form, orally in a meeting, or may be audiotaped
(4)   Information shared during the end of shift report should include:
      (a)   Basic identifying information about each patient-name and current diagnosis
      (b)   Current health status to include changes in medical condition and patient's response to medical therapy
      (c)   Current orders (especially newly changed orders or new medications)
      (d)   Diagnostic tests or schedule surgeries
      (e)   Summary of each newly admitted patient including his or her diagnosis, age, plan of treatment, and general condition

Medical Record Forms

SF 600 - chronological record of medical care

SF 511 - chronological inpatient record of TPR, BP and weight

DD Form 792, 24 hour I & O worksheet
(1)   Chronological record of intake (front side of SF 511) -
      (a)   Oral intake
      (b)   IV intake
      (c)   irrigation
      (d)   Blood products
(2)   Chronological record of output (back side of SF 511) -
      (a)   Urine
      (b)   Nasogastric
      (c)   Chest
      (d)   Emesis
      (e)   Stools
      (f)   Other

SF 558 - Used instead of SF 600 in emergency rooms

SF 510, Nursing notes

Other forms
(1)   Lab slips
      (a)   Miscellaneous
      (b)   Chemistry

         (c)   Urinalysis
         (d)   Hematology
         (e)   Culture

(2)   Special procedure forms
         (a)   SF 519-B x-ray request
         (b)   SF 520 EKG request
         (c)   Be sure to write the provider's name as well as the name and phone number of the ward/clinic sending the request on all request forms!

(3)   Sick-Call forms (Refer to LP Perform Medical Screening C191W017)
         (a)   DA Form 5181-R Screening of acute medical care
         (b)   DD Form 689 Individual sick slip

Introduction to Composite Health Care System (CHCS)

The Composite Health Care System (CHCS) provides worldwide automated medical information system support to all MTFs in providing comprehensive, high quality health care to uniformed service personnel, retirees and dependents.

Functions performed by CHCS

(1)   CHCS serves more than 9 million beneficiaries of the U.S. military health care worldwide

(2)   CHCS is installed in more than 700 DOD hospitals and clinics providing health care to the men and women of the armed services and their dependents, veterans, and the retired military community

(3)   CHCS:
         (a)   Shorter waits for patients
         (b)   Faster reporting of diagnostic test results
         (c)   Improved use of the medical and professional resources
         (d)   Significant improvements in the quality of patient care

(4)   CHCS Functions:
         (a)   Patient registration, admission, disposition, and transfer
         (b)   Inpatient activity documentation
         (c)   Outpatient administration data
         (d)   Appointment scheduling
         (e)   Laboratory
         (f)   Drug/laboratory test interaction
         (g)   Quality assurance
         (h)   Radiology
         (i)   Clinical dietetic administration
         (j)   Pharmacy
         (k)   Results reporting and order entry
         (l)   Ad Hoc reporting
         (m)   Managed Care
         (n)   Interfaces to 40 other clinical and administrative systems

Benefits to Medical Professionals

(1)   For the health care professional, CHCS saves staff time and increases job performance and satisfaction
(2)   CHCS offers medical professionals:
    (a)   Immediate notification of test results
    (b)   Improved drug inventories, allowing pharmacies to monitor shelf life and drug quantities
    (c)   Reduced paperwork
    (d)   Improved accuracy of laboratory and radiology results
    (e)   Easy access to complete patient care information and administrative data
    (f)   Better quality control with enhanced capabilities for monitoring productivity and quality assurance data
    (g)   Increased productivity and utilization management control
    (h)   Improved communication with administrative staff and other health care professionals
    (i)   Improved clinic administration
    (j)   Improved documentation and accountability for patients' medication orders
    (k)   Better utilization of staff resources due to improved scheduling
    (l)   Systematic tracking of a patient's treatment course

Cost Benefits
(1)   CHCS reduces costs by eliminating duplication and tracking of data to assist in determining the most successful medical strategies
(2)   CHCS provides:
    (a)   Immediate access to information, allowing prompt evaluation of cost effectiveness and resource utilization
    (b)   Systematic tracking of a patient's treatment course, thereby reducing duplicative services, tests, and drug orders
    (c)   Treatment pattern comparisons, helping providers to determine the most successful and cost-effective clinical protocols
    (d)   Improved data collection for outcome studies

Benefits to Patients
(1)   On the patient level, CHCS increases quality of care by providing complete, accurate, and secure information about patients and their care
(2)   CHCS means:
    (a)   Authorized users can immediately access private, personal medical records, thus facilitating appropriate patient care and saving lives in emergency situations
    (b)   Improved access to health care services due to better scheduling and resource utilization
    (c)   Fewer repeated tests and examinations thanks to improved reporting and data management
    (d)   More responsive scheduling and handling of appointments

(e)   More personal service from MTF staff and health care providers

(f)   Improved health care professional/patient relationships

(g)   Shorter waits for pharmacy services

(h)   Fewer delays in receiving radiology and lab tests and results

(i)   Constantly updated and accurate patient registration information

(j)   Greater patient satisfaction with service and results

(k)   Facilitates enrollment to TRICARE programs

TERMINAL LEARNING OBJECTIVE

Give the necessary medical equipment in a holding or ward setting, provide casualty care as part of an integrated team in a Minimal Care Ward by administering medication to a casualty without causing further injury or illness.

Drug effects-mechanism of action

(1)   Predictable chemical reaction-how the drug works
(2)   Changes the physiological activity of the body as the drug bonds chemically at a specific site called a receptor site
(3)   Mechanism of actions of drugs include
        (a)   Drugs that fit the receptor sites well with a good chemical response are called „agonists"
        (b)   Drugs that attach at a receptor site and become chemically inactive with no drug response is called an „antagonist"
        (c)   Drugs that attach at a receptor site and produce a slight chemical reaction are called „partial agonists"

Drug actions

(1)   Therapeutic effects
        (a)   Expected positive effect of drug
        (b)   Single medication may have many therapeutic effects such as aspirin which is an analgesic, reduces inflammation, reduces fever and reduces clot formation
        (c)   Some drugs have very specific effects such as antihypertensive medications have a therapeutic effect of controlling high blood pressure. Antibiotics treat bacterial infections.
(2)   Side effects
        (a)   Unintended secondary effects
        (b)   May or may not be harmful to the patient
        (c)   Side effects of a drug may outweigh the benefits
        (d)   Patients may stop taking a drug because of unpleasant side effects, i.e. codeine prescribed to control coughing but causes constipation.
(3)   Toxic effects
        (a)   Caused by intake of high doses of medications, ingestion of drugs not intended to be ingested, such as topical medications, or when a drug accumulates in the system due to impaired metabolism or excretion
        (b)   May be lethal, depending on the action of the drug
        (c)   Usually seen in accidental poisonings and intentional drug overdoses i.e., intentional ingestion or accidental administration of a large amount of a narcotic may cause severe respiratory depression and death.
(4)   Allergic Reactions
        (a)   Unpredictable response to a drug
        (b)   May be mild or severe

(c)   Mild allergic reactions include hives, rash, pruritus (itching of the skin), rhinitis (stuffy, runny nose) and wheezing.

(d)   Severe or anaphylactic reactions are characterized by sudden constriction of the bronchiolar muscles, swelling the throat, severe wheezing and shortness of breath. Without immediate life saving measures, this reaction progresses rapidly and death can occur within minutes.

(e)   Always ask patient about allergies to medications. Check unconscious patients for a medical alert bracelet or medal indicating a medication allergy prior to administering medications

(5)   Drug tolerance and dependence

(a)   Occurs when the patient receives the same drug for long periods of time and requires higher doses to produce the same effect.

(b)   For example, patients who take pain medications over a long period of time may develop a tolerance for the drug and require higher doses to achieve the same effect.

(6)   Drug interactions:

(a)   One drug modifies the action of another drug. Drug interactions are common in patients who take many medications

(b)   A drug may potentiate or diminish the action of other drugs

(c)   May alter the way a drug is absorbed, metabolized or eliminated from the body

(d)   Drug interactions may or may not be desirable. For example, combining alcohol with other central nervous system depressants is not desirable. Combining diuretics and vasodilators act together to lower blood pressure in a desirable way.

Routes of drug administration

Non-parenteral medication administration

(1)   Drugs are introduced into the body by different routes, each serving a specific purpose

(2)   Oral administration of medications is the most common method

(a)   Advantages

     (i)   Convenience

     (ii)   Economy

     (iii)   The drug need not be absolutely pure or sterile

     (iv)   A wide variety of dosage forms are available

(b)   Oral medications include tablets, capsules, liquids, and suspensions

(c)   Disadvantages include

     (i)   Inability of some patients to swallow

     (ii)   Slow absorption

     (iii)   Partial or complete destruction by the digestive system

(d)   Other routes associated closely with oral administration

(i)   Sublingual - under the mouth
(ii)   Buccal - The drug is placed between the cheek and gum and is quickly absorbed directly into the blood stream

(3)   Inhalation
    (a)   The introduction of medications through the respiratory system in the form of a gas, vapor, or powder
    (b)   Divided into three major types:
        (i)   Vaporization - the drug is changed from a liquid or solid to a gas or vapor by the use of heat, such as steam inhalation
        (ii)   Gas inhalation- almost entirely restricted to anesthesia
        (iii)   Nebulization - the drug is nebulized into minute droplets by the use of compressed gas

(4)   Topical Ointments
    (a)   Examples of topical preparations
        (i)   Creams
        (ii)   Lotions
        (iii)   Shampoos
    (b)   Topical application serves two purposes:
        (i)   Local effect-the drug is intended to relieve itching, burning, or other skin conditions without being absorbed into the bloodstream and
        (ii)   Systemic effect-the drug is absorbed through the skin into the bloodstream.
        (iii)   Example: Nitroglycerin paste

(5)   Suppositories
    (a)   Rectal is preferred to the oral route when patient is
        (i)   Nauseated or vomiting
        (ii)   Unconscious, uncooperative, or mentally incapable
    (b)   Vaginal suppositories, creams, or tablets are examples of vaginal preparations that are inserted into the vagina to produce a local effect

Parenteral medications are those introduced by injection

(1)   All drugs used by this route must be
    (a)   Pure
    (b)   Sterile
    (c)   Pyrogen-free (pyrogens are products of the growth of microorganisms)
    (d)   Liquid state
(2)   Several types of parenteral administration
    (a)   Subcutaneous
        (i)   The agent is injected just below the skin's cutaneous layers
        (ii)   Example: Insulin
    (b)   Intradermal

    (i) The drug is injected within the dermis
    (ii) Example: Purified protein derivative (PPD)
  (c) Intramuscular
    (i) The drug is injected into the muscle
    (ii) Example: Procaine penicillin G
  (d) Intravenous
    (i) The drug is introduced directly into the vein
    (ii) Example: Intravenous fluids / antibiotics
  (e) Intrathecal/intraspinal
    (i) The drug is introduced into the subarachnoid space of the spinal column

Bulk and Unit Dose Medications

Bulk drugs

(1) Commonly called floor stock or clinic stock
(2) Description - large quantity of drug from which individual medication dose is removed
(3) Storage guidelines
  (a) Once individual dosage is removed, it can NEVER be returned to bulk container
  (b) Individual dosage drawn from bulk drug container will be disposed of IAW local SOP
  (c) Some medications require controlled temperature storage ranges

Unit dose

(1) Description - single dose of a drug in a tablet, capsule, liquid, or injectable form that is prepackaged by the pharmaceutical company or pharmacy
(2) Storage guidelines
  (a) Normally found in medication cart
  (b) If still in original wrapper/unused condition, can be returned to medication cart/storage

Internal and topical (external) medications must be stored separately to prevent accidental use of the inappropriate medication

(1) Injectable
(2) Ointments
(3) Tablets are stored on separate shelves

Specific medications kept in secured (limited access) area

(1) All narcotics
(2) All medications with abuse potential, e.g., diazepam (Valium)
(3) All pre-filled hypodermic needles and syringes

Guidelines and Principles

General guidelines

(1)   Check the physician's/PA orders
(2)   Wash hands prior to touching any medication
(3)   Five patient rights
    (a)   Right patient - verify patient's identity by comparing the patient's medical record, provider's orders, and the medical bracelet (hospital) or ask patient to state full name
    (b)   Right medication - compare provider's orders, medication sheet, and medication label
    (c)   Right dose - ensure amount of medication ordered by the provider is measured correctly (i.e., graduated medicine cup, syringe, number of tablets, number of milligrams, etc.)
    (d)   Right time - administer medications at the prescribed time as per provider's orders
    (e)   Right route - administer medication via the route specified in the provider's order (i.e., PO, IM, IV, etc.)
(4)   Check medical records, allergy bands, medic-alert tags and ask patient for medication allergies

Principles of Medication Administration

(1)   Only administer medication that you have prepared or received from the pharmacy as unit dose
(2)   Be familiar with all potential medication effects, both therapeutic and non-therapeutic. This information can be found in the:
    (a)   Manufacturer's medication insert that accompanies prepackaged medications
    (b)   Local SOP
    (c)   If available, Physicians Desk Reference (PDR) or RN's Drug Book

CAUTION: If there is any doubt about administering a medication, check with supervisor, nurse, physician, or pharmacist.

(3)   Administration route and time will be followed IAW provider's orders

WARNING: NEVER alter medication dosage ordered by physician!

(4)   If in doubt about medication dose, time, administration route, or if a medication is missing, check with supervisor, nurse, physician, PA or pharmacist
    (a)   MD/PA's order and medication label DO NOT match exactly
    (b)   Illegible medication label; return to pharmacy or follow local SOP
(5)   Check all medications label 3 times to ensure that the correct medication is being prepared for administration

        (a)   When removing the medication or container from the storage area

        (b)   When preparing the medication dose

        (c)   When returning the container to the storage area

(6)   Check the expiration date of the medication

(7)   Handle only one medication at a time

(8)   While administering medication, do not perform other duties (i.e., obtain vital signs, dressing changes)

(9)   Prepare the prescribed dose of medication

        (a)   Tablet or capsules - transfer the prescribed dose of tablets or capsules to the medicine cup or if unit dose- open the package and give directly to the patient

        (b)   Liquids - pour the prescribed dose of liquid medication into the medicine cup. Small amounts of liquid medication should be drawn up in a syringe

        (c)   Powders - pour the correct dose of powdered or granulated medication into the medicine cup

                (i)   Pour the required amount of water or juice into a paper cup

                (ii)   Reconstitute the medication at the patient's bedside

WARNING: Never directly touch oral medications. Some medications can be absorbed through the skin, also the medication will become contaminated.

                (iii)   The medic may assist the patient in taking the medication if the patient is physically unable

WARNING: DO NOT administer oral medications to patients with a decreased level of consciousness. Check with supervisor for instructions.

CAUTION: Positive patient ID required prior to administering medication.

(10)   Patient Identification

        (a)   Patient Identification (Hospital)

                (i)   Be sure the patient has received and wears an identification band

                (ii)   Check the information on the band to see that it is correct

                (iii)   Check the tag on the bed or wall and door, and make sure the patient is properly identified

                (iv)   Ask the patient to state his/her name

                (v)   Check patient ID band for medication allergies and other pertinent information

                (vi)   In a hospital environment, have patients return to their bedside to receive medication

        (b)   Patient Identification (Clinic)

                (i)   Have patient state name

(ii)   Ask patient if he/she has any allergies to
         medications

Dosage

Systems of drug measurement (definitions)

(1)   Metric System
         (a)   Decimal system, each basic unit of measure is organized
                 into units of 10
         (b)   Basic units of measure are the meter (length), the liter
                 (volume), and the gram (weight)
         (c)   Small or large letters are used to designate the basic units:
                 (i)   Gram = g or GM
                 (ii)   Liter = l or L
         (d)   Small letters are abbreviations for subdivisions of major
                 units:
                 (i)   Milligram = mg
                 (ii)   Milliliter = ml
(2)   Apothecary System
         (a)   One of oldest systems of measurement
         (b)   Seldom used, but some companies include apothecary
                 measure in addition to the metric
         (c)   Basic units of measure include grains (weight), and
                 minims, drams, and ounces (volume)
         (d)   Measurements are approximates and a 10% variance has
                 become acceptable in preparation and administration of
                 most medications
         (e)   Uses roman numerals and fractions
                 (i)   ss = ½
                 (ii)   Abbreviation or symbol for a unit of measure is
                          written before the amount of quantity
(3)   Household measurements
         (a)   Familiar to most people
         (b)   Used when more accurate systems of measure are
                 unnecessary
         (c)   Basic units of measure include drops, teaspoons,
                 tablespoons, cups, and glass for volume; and ounces and
                 pounds for weight

Dosage

(1)   A dose is the amount of medication to be administered
(2)   Posology is the study of dosage and the criteria that influence it
(3)   United States Pharmacopeia and National Formulary (USP-NF)
        states the doses given are the average therapeutic doses or "usual
        adult doses"
(4)   The following terms are used in connection with doses:
         (a)   Therapeutic dose

i

            (i)   Amount needed to produce the desired therapeutic effect

            (ii)   Also referred to as „usual adult dose„

            (iii)   Calculated on an average adult about 24 years old, weighing approximately 150 pounds

(b)   Dosage range

            (i)   The range between the MINIMUM amount of drug and the MAXIMUM amount of drug required to produce the desired effect

            (ii)   Many drugs, such as antibiotics, require large initial doses that are later tapered to smaller amounts

            (iii)   MINIMUM dose, the least amount of drug required to produce a therapeutic effect

            (iv)   MAXIMUM dose, the largest amount of drug that can be given without reaching the toxic effect

            (v)   TOXIC dose, the least amount of drug that will produce symptoms of poisoning

            (vi)   Minimum lethal dose - The least amount of drug than can produce death

Factors Affecting Dosage

(1)   Many factors that affect the dose, method of administration, and frequency of the dose

(2)   Although a physician prescribes the amount to be given, you need to know how and why these quantities are determined

(3)   Two primary factors that determine or influence the dose are age and weight

(4)   **Age** is the most common factor that influences the amount of drug to be given

            (a)   An infant would require much less than an adult

            (b)   Elderly patients may require more or less than the average dose, depending upon the action of the drug and the condition of the patient

(5)   **Weight** has a more direct bearing on the dose than any other factor, especially in the calculation of pediatric doses

(6)   Other factors that influence dosage are:

            (a)   Genetic make-up: The genetic structure of the individual may cause peculiar reactions to medications in some patients

            (b)   Habitual use: Some patients must take medications chronically, causing their bodies to build up tolerance to the drug. This tolerance may require larger doses than their initial doses to obtain the same therapeutic effect.

            (c)   Time of administration: Therapeutic effect may be altered depending upon time of administration. Example: Before or after meals.

            (d)   Mode of administration: This has a definite impact on the dose. Example: Injections

Principles

Patient observation

(1)   Remain with patient until medication is swallowed completely, injected, or applied topically

(2)   If patient refuses medication
- (a)   Remove medication from the patient's room
- (b)   Report the omission to the nurse/supervisor
- (c)   Offer the medication again in five minutes
- (d)   If refused a second time, record the omission per SOP and document the reason for the omission in the nursing notes

CAUTION: DO NOT leave medications at the patient's bedside without a specific physician's order to do so.

(3)   Observe for medication effects and/or side effects
- (a)   Medical History
  - (i)   Before administering medications, review the patient's medical history for possible indications or contraindications for medication therapy
  - (ii)   Disease or illness may place patient at risk for adverse medication effects
  - (iii)   Long-term health problems or surgical history may require medications
- (b)   History of Allergies
  - (i)   Allergic to medication
  - (ii)   Food allergies should be documented
  - (iii)   If patient is allergic to shellfish, they may be sensitive to any product containing iodine such as Betadine or dyes used in radiological testing
- (c)   Medication History
  - (i)   Length of time drug has been taken
  - (ii)   Current dosage schedule
  - (iii)   Any ill effects experienced
  - (iv)   Drug data: action, purpose, normal dosage, routes, side effects and nursing implications for administration and monitoring

(4)   If the patient has an adverse reaction. (Rash, itching, and nausea/vomiting/diarrhea are common examples of adverse reactions.)

WARNING: Anaphylaxis is the most severe form of adverse reaction to a medication.
- (a)   Stop dosage immediately
- (b)   Assess patient's airway, breathing, circulation
- (c)   Inform nurse/physician on duty immediately

Medical documentation

    (1)   Record administration of medication IAW SOP. Minimum information needed is
- (a)   Name of medication given
- (b)   Dosage of medication
- (c)   Time given
- (d)   Route of administration
- (e)   Patient's reaction (effects/side effects)
- (f)   Name of person who administered medication

    (2)   Record the omission of a medication on the appropriate medical forms whenever a scheduled medication is not administered IAW local SOP

Medication Errors

Any event that causes the patient to receive inappropriate drug therapy (medications) or failing to receive appropriate drug therapy (medications)

Can be made by anyone involved in the prescribing (MD/PA), transcribing of the order, preparing and dispensing (pharmacist, RN, 91W) or administering the medication (RN, LPN, 91W)

Strict adherence to the five „rights" of medication administration helps to prevent errors

Errors should be acknowledged as soon as they are discovered or known to have happened and reported immediately to the appropriate people for patient follow-up

Professional and ethical obligations to your patients mandate that you report all medication errors

TERMINAL LEARNING OBJECTIVE

Give the necessary medical equipment in a holding or ward setting. You are providing casualty care as part of an integrated team in a Minimal Care Ward.

Facts related to the pain experience
Pain is the body's defense mechanism that indicates the person is experiencing a problem.

Classic definition of pain: Pain is an abstract concept which refers to a personal, private sensation of hurt, a harmful stimulus which signals current or impending tissue damage, and a pattern of responses which operate to protect the organism.

Leading nursing definition: Pain is whatever the experiencing person says it is, existing whenever he/she says it does.

Origins of Pain
Physical Origin
(1)   Cutaneous pain
     (a)   Superficial, usually involves the skin or subcutaneous tissue
     (b)   Example: A paper cut that produces sharp pain with a burning sensation
(2)   Somatic pain
     (a)   Diffuse or scattered and originates in tendons, ligaments, bones, blood vessels, and nerves
     (b)   Example: Strong pressure on a bone or damage to tissue that occurs with a sprain causes deep somatic pain
(3)   Visceral pain
     (a)   Poorly localized and originates in body organs (thorax, cranium, abdomen)
     (b)   Visceral pain usually presents as referred pain, which is perceived in an area distant from the point of origin
     (c)   Example: Pain associated with a myocardial infarction is frequently referred to the neck, shoulder, or left arm

Psychogenic pain
(1)   Physical cause for the pain cannot be identified
(2)   Pain can be just as intense as pain that results from a physical origin
     Responses to Pain
     Physiologic (involuntary)
(1)   Sympathetic response- moderate and superficial
     (a)   Increased blood pressure, pulse, and respirations
     (b)   Pupil dilation
     (c)   Muscle tension and rigidity
     (d)   Pallor
     (e)   Increased adrenaline output
     (f)   Increased glucose
(2)   Parasympathetic response to severe and deep pain
     (a)   Nausea and vomiting
     (b)   Fainting and unconsciousness

(c)	Decreased blood pressure
(d)	Decreased pulse rate
(e)	Prostration - a condition of extreme exhaustion and inability to exert oneself further, as in heat prostration or nervous prostration
(f)	Rapid and irregular breathing

Behavioral

(1)   Moving away from painful stimuli
(2)   Grimacing, moaning, and crying
(3)   Restlessness
(4)   Protecting the painful area and refusing to move

Affective

(1)   Examples - exaggerated weeping and restlessness, withdrawal, anxiety, depression, and fear
(2)   Person's past experience with pain and sociocultural background play an important role in emotional responses to pain
(3)   Emotions tend to intensify the reactions to pain
(4)   Explains why similar circumstances causes a different pain responses in different groups of people

Acute Versus Chronic Pain

(1)   Acute pain
    (a)   Generally rapid onset
    (b)   Varies in intensity from mild to severe
    (c)   May last for a brief period up to a period of 6 months
    (d)   Protective in nature, warns of tissue damage or organic disease
    (e)   Once underlying cause is resolved, pain disappears
    (f)   Examples: pricked finger, sore throat, post surgical pain
(2)   Chronic pain
    (a)   Last 6 months or longer and interferes with normal functioning
    (b)   May be limited, intermittent or persistent

Factors Affecting the Pain Experience

Culture

(1)   Cultures vary in what is an acceptable response to pain
(2)   An assessment of the cultural influences of:
    (a)   The meaning of the pain event
    (b)   Ways in which patient choose to demonstrate and cope with the pain experience
    (c)   Responsibilities in pain relief

Religion

(1)   Religion can effect patient's views on their pain experience
(2)   Some see pain as a purifying experience. This becomes a sense of strength for them. these patients might refuse pain medications.
(3)   Pain might be viewed as a punishment from God. These patients might become angry and resentful.

Anxiety and other stressors

(1)   Anxiety leads to muscle tension and fatigue which can also increase pain
        intensity
(2)   Factors which may increase anxiety:
        (a)   Strange environment in the hospital
        (b)   Support people not available
        (c)   Fear of the unknown

Past pain experience
(1)   Whether the patient has experienced pain in the past and qualities of that
        experience profoundly affect new pain experiences
(2)   Some patients have never known severe pain and have no fear of pain.
        Patients who have had severe pain without adequate pain relief may have
        increase sensitivity to pain

Components of Pain Assessment

Characteristics of pain (PQRST)

(1)   Provokes pain
        (a)   Aggravating factors
        (i)   Question the patient on what makes the pain increase
        (ii)   Example: "Does your pain become worse upon exertion?„
        (b)   Alleviating factors
        (i)   Ask patient to describe what makes pain go away or lessen.
        (ii)   Determine what pain relief methods have worked in the past. For
                how long these pain relief methods used?
(2)   Quality
        (a)   Encourage the patient to descriptive words to describe his/her pain
        (b)   Examples: sharp, stabbing, pressure, dull, aching
(3)   Radiation (Location)
        (a)   Instruct the patient to point the area of pain. Patients with chronic or
                visceral pain might have difficulty localizing specific area.
        (b)   Clearly document areas of pain. Utilize a diagram of the body to be
                more specific if needed.
(4)   Severity
        (a)   Since pain is subjective, it is very important to have patients rate the
                pain they are experiencing. This becomes extremely important when
                assessing the effectiveness of pain medications.
        (b)   Various scales may be used. One example is a 0-10 scale:
        0   No Pain
        1
        2   Mild Pain
        3
        4
        5   Moderate Pain
        6
        7   Severe Pain
        8
        9

10   As bad as it can be Pain
(c)   Ask patient to rate pain at various stages
(i)   At its worse
(ii)   At its least
(iii)   After pain medication
(5)   Time
(a)   Duration
(i)   Ask how long the patient has been experiencing the pain
(ii)   If pain is intermittent, ask how long the pain lasts and how often does pain occur
(b)   Chronology
(i)   Have the patient describe how the pain first began
(ii)   Question if the pain has change since the onset
(iii)   Identify if the pain is worsening or improving
(iv)   Is the pain intermittent or constant?
(6)   Associated phenomena
(a)   Identify if there were any factors that seem to relate consistently to the pain
(b)   Examples: Increased anxiety before pain begins

Physiological responses

(1)   Sympathetic stimulation – occur with acute pain
(2)   Parasympathetic stimulation - with prolonged severe pain
(3)   Responses to watch: Vital signs, skin color, perspiration, pupil size, nausea, muscle tension, anxiety

Behavioral Responses

(1)   Posture, gross motor activities
(a)   Assess if the patient guards an area
(b)   Does the patient make frequent position changes?
(c)   Posture and gross motor activities increased in acute pain, might be absent with chronic pain
(2)   Facial features - Does the patient have a pinched look? Are there facial grimaces? Look of fatigue?
(3)   Verbal expression - Does patient sigh, moan, scream, cry, repeat same words?

Methods used in the Relief of Pain

Non-pharmocologic relief measures

(1)   Distraction
(a)   Techniques for distraction
(i)   Visual - Staring at an object or spot and describing it in detail, reading or watching television
(ii)   Auditory - listening to music
(iii)   Tactile/Kinesthetic – Holding or stroking a loved one, pet, or toy, rocking back and forth, slow breathing

	(iv)	Project Distraction – Playing a games, creative work, writing in a journal
	(b)	Requires the patient to focus on something other than the pain
	(c)	Best used before the pain starts or becomes moderate to severe. Is not to be used as the only intervention for severe pain. Can be used as adjuvant treatment.
(2)		Imagery – example of mind-body interaction-concentrates on an image that involves one or all of the senses , gradually becomes less aware of the pain. Does not work as the only intervention for severe pain.
(3)		Relaxation - techniques to relieve anxiety and reduce stress. Includes listening to music while taking slow deep breaths and consciously relaxing each muscle group. Should be utilized early in the pain experience. Patient should practice technique.

Pharmocologic

(1)		Non-narcotic analgesics (aspirin, Tylenol, NSAIDS)
	(a)	Used for mild to moderate pain
	(b)	Works best on muscle and joint pain.
	(c)	Produces analgesia at the peripheral nervous system.
	(d)	Major Side-effects: Nausea, vomiting, increased bleeding tendencies.
(2)		Narcotic analgesic (morphine, codiene, demerol)
	(a)	Used for severe pain.
	(b)	In sufficient dose, considered capable of relieving pain, in most cases
	(c)	Analgesia produced at the central nervous system
	(d)	Major side-effect: Respiratory depression, sedation and addiction
(3)		Adjuvant analgesics (antidepressants, anticonvulsants)
	(a)	Used usually in combination with opioids especially when there is a neurologic component as one of the causes of the pain.
	(b)	Mechanism of action not clearly understood, may block pain transmission or may suppress abnormal nerve endings from injury to nerve tissue (anticonvulsant).

91W Solider Medic' s Role in Pain Management

Obtain a thorough baseline pain assessment

Assess pt's beliefs and misconceptions regarding pain management

Provide patient education regarding pain management regime

(1)   Assure the patient that every step will be taken to treat their pain effectively. Do not let the patient think he/she is being left alone to DEAL with the pain.

(2)   Correct any misconceptions regarding pain medication that the patient might have. Reinforce information regarding newly prescribed medication.

In the hospitalized patient, document the patient's response to the pain medication. This is very important for the ongoing accurate assessment of the patient's pain.

When administering narcotic analgesia, monitor for signs and symptoms of overdose, especially respiratory depression and severe sedation. Obtain baseline respirations before administering medication.

Inform health care team if pain management regime is not effective

TERMINAL LEARNING OBJECTIVE

Given a patient/casualty with known symptoms the soldier medic will be able to identify and use available drugs.

Sources of Drugs

Plants
- (1)   Belladonna
- (2)   Opium

Animals
- (1)   Heparin
- (2)   Insulin

Minerals
- (1)   Iodine
- (2)   Iron (Fe + 2)

Microorganisms
- (1)   Antibiotics--penicillin, tetracycline
- (2)   Vaccines

Synthetics
- (1)   Aspirin
- (2)   Acetaminophen

Use of Drugs

Maintain health
- (1)   Treatment of disease--antibiotics and chemotherapeutic (anticancer) agents are commonly used in medicine today
- (2)   To relieve symptoms--drugs which act to relieve symptoms but do not cure the patient. Instead, they help to make the patient more comfortable in order for the patient to work or function.

Prevent disease
- (1)   Immunization--vaccines and toxoids are used to prevent disease
- (2)   Nutrition--vitamins and minerals

Diagnose disease-
Radiopharmaceuticals are used to diagnose many diseases

Prevent pregnancy

Factors that Affect the Desired Effect of a Drug

Age-
As a general rule, the very young and the very old require smaller doses than the average adult

34

Size-
    (1)   Weight--obese or larger patients may require a
                higher dose of medication to achieve the same
                effect than a thin or smaller patient
    (2)   Surface area--this takes into account both the
                patients height and weight for the determining of
                the proper dose of medication. This method is
                more accurate than using just the patient's weight
                and is routinely used for antineoplastic (cancer)
                medications

Sex-
Females have more adipose (fat) cells than males, in
proportion to their body weight. As a result, females may
need higher doses of fat-soluble drugs to achieve the same
effects. The utilization and metabolism of various hormones
is also effected by gender.

Time of administration-
Time of day a medication is administered may alter the
amount of drug that is absorbed. For example, many
antibiotics are have a higher degree of bioavailability if taken
before meals (on an empty stomach), while some actually
work better if taken after a meal

Drug interactions-
Interaction between two or more drugs may affect the overall
effectiveness of each drug
    (1)   Synergistic--the joint action of drugs. The
                combined effect is greater then the sum of the
                individual effects. (1 + 1 = 3)
    (2)   Additive--the combined effect is equal to the sum
                of the effects of the individual agents. (1 + 1 = 2)
                (i.e., 1 Aspirin and 1 Acetaminophen given
                together for fever.)
    (3)   Antagonistic--the combined effect is actually less
                then the action of either agent (1+1=0)

Tolerance-
After taking a medication for some time, a patient may
require a larger dose to obtain the desired effect (opiates,
cocaine, amphetamines, and barbiturates). This is
especially true for narcotic analgesics. Cross-tolerance--the
use of one drug can cause tolerance to another--addicts can
develop tolerance to sedatives and anesthetics

Genetic factors-
Different ethnic groups may metabolize certain drugs at
different rates

Physical condition of patient-
Weak, ill, or debilitated patients may require less medication. Patients in severe pain may require a higher dose of analgesics to relieve the pain

Routes of administration-
Route of administration may determine the rate of absorption, or the amount of drug that is metabolized

Psychological condition of the patient-
In some cases, if a patient believes that the medication will work, the patient may obtain a positive clinical response. This is termed the placebo effect

Routes of Administration

Oral
- (1)   Tablet; capsule; liquid
- (2)   Usually taken for systemic effect
- (3)   Must pass through stomach and be absorbed
- (4)   Delayed onset of action

Sublingual
- (1)   Dissolved under tongue
- (2)   Taken for systemic effect
- (3)   Rapid onset of action
- (4)   Avoids gut

Buccal
- (1)   Dissolved in pouch of cheek
- (2)   Taken for systemic effect
- (3)   More rapid onset of action than oral route, but less than sublingual route
- (4)   Avoids gut

Rectal
- (1)   Cream, suppository, or liquid
- (2)   Used for local and systemic effect
- (3)   Useful in unconscious or pediatric patients

Vaginal/urethral
- (1)   Cream or suppository
- (2)   Used for local effect
- (3)   Should not irritate tissue
- (4)   May be absorbed

Inhalation
- (1)   Sprays, gases, powders
- (2)   Used for local or systemic effect
- (3)   May be administered nasally or orally

Topical
- (1)   Sprays, creams, powders, gels, ointments, patches
- (2)   Used for local or systemic effect

Parenteral
- (1)   Advantages
  - (a)   By-pass the G.I. tract

(b)   Rapid onset of action
(c)   Prolonged action, depending on vehicle
(d)   Used for local or systemic effects
(2)   Disadvantages
     (a)   Painful to the patient
     (b)   Inconvenient
     (c)   Once medication is administered, you can't recover the drug
     (d)   May expose nursing staff to blood or body fluids
(3)   Types of parenteral routes:
     (a)   Intravenous (I.V.)
          (i)   Most rapid onset
          (ii)   Drug injected directly into vein
     (b)   Intramuscular (I.M.)
          (i)   Drug injected deep into muscle
          (ii)   If aqueous base, absorption is rapid, but slower than the intravenous route
          (iii)   If oil base, absorption is slow
     (c)   Intradermal (I.D.)
          (i)   Drug injected into dermal layer of the skin
          (ii)   Used for diagnostic tests
     (d)   Subcutaneous (SQ/SC)
          (i)   Drug injected into the fatty layer below skin, but not into the muscle
          (ii)   Route is slower than the IM route, because the subcutaneous tissue is less vascular than the muscular tissue
          (iii)   Must be nonirritating or it may cause tissue necrosis
     (e)   Spinal (Intrathecal, Epidural, & Caudal) - Drug injected into or near the spinal cord

Adverse Reactions to Drugs

Direct toxicity
(1)   Blood dyscrasias--damaging to the components of the blood (RBCs, WBCs, platelets etc.)
(2)   Hepatotoxicity--damaging to the liver (liver is organ which detoxifies drugs)
(3)   Nephrotoxicity--damaging to the kidney (kidney eliminates water soluble toxic agents)
(4)   Teratogenicity--causes birth defects (drugs can cross the placental barrier. Fetus most

susceptible in first trimester of the female
pregnancy. Referred to as teratogenic.)

Allergic reactions--hypersensitivity
    (1)   Caused by prior exposure to agent or similar drug-
sensitization
    (2)   Reaction varies from rash to anaphylaxis

Side effects
    (1)   Most drugs affect more than one system
    (2)   Some side effects are minor, others are so
distressing as to cause the patient to stop taking
the drug (i.e. vomiting, diarrhea)

Drug dependence
    (1)   Psychological--patient convinced that he/she has
a need for the drug. The mind tells the patient that
they must have the drug to function normally
    (2)   Physiological--body develops a need for the drug,
if drug is taken away, patient goes through
withdrawal, tremors, nausea, vomiting, and
convulsions. The body exhibits physical signs of
the need for the drug. The classic example is a
narcotic addict

Medications for use by the Soldier Medic

Oral medications
For fever and pain
(a) Acetaminophen-nonnarcotic analgesic and antipyretic
    (i)   Indications
        *   Mild pain
        *   Fever
    (ii) Contraindications- patients with hypersensitivity to
the drug
    (iii) Side effects - rare
        *   May cause liver damage in high doses or
unsupervised long-term use
        *   Patients should be warned that excessive
ingestion of alcohol while using
acetaminophen could result in severe liver
damage.
    (iv) Dosage
        *   Adults: 325-650 mg P.O. (by mouth) every 4-
6 hours or 1 Gram every 6-8 hours as
needed for fever or mild pain
        *   May also be given as a rectal suppository-
650 mg every 4-6 hours as needed for mild
pain or fever
        *   Maximum daily dose (24 hours) should not
exceed 4 grams.

(v) Considerations
   * Use cautiously in patients with history of chronic alcohol use-liver damage has occurred with therapeutic doses
   * Many over the counter products contain acetaminophen. Be aware of this when calculating total daily dose
(vi) Common brand name: Tylenol
(b) Ibuprofen-nonsteroidal anti-inflammatory drug (NSAID)
   (i) Indications
      * Mild to moderate pain relief to include headaches (analgesia)
      * fever reduction (antipyretic)
   (ii) Contraindications
      * Patients with hypersensitivity to the drug
      * Patients with known ulcer disease
   (iii) Side effects – Increases bleeding time for 8 hours
      * Gastrointestinal (GI) pain
      * Nausea
      * Occult gastrointestinal bleeding
   (iv) Dosage
      * For mild to moderate pain 400-800 mg P.O. every 6-8 hours
      * For fever, 200-800 mg P.O. every 6-8 hours
      * Maximum daily dose (24 hours) 3200 mg.
   (v) Considerations
      * Take with meals or milk to reduce GI side effects
      * Do not use with aspirin or alcohol, which may increase risk of GI reactions
      * Serious GI bleeding can occur in patients taking NSAIDs despite absence of symptoms
      * Patients should be taught the signs and symptoms of GI bleeding (dark, „tarry„ stools, „coffee ground„ or bloody emesis) and instructed to notify the MD/PA immediately if they occur.
   (vi) Common brand names
      * Motrin
      * Advil
      * Nuprin

For cough, colds, and sinus allergies
(a) **Actifed**- Combination of two drugs-psuedoephedrine HCL (decongestant) 60 mg and Tripolidine HCL (antihistamine) 2.5 mg.
   (i) Indications
      * Colds
      * Nasal congestion
      * Seasonal allergy symptoms

(ii) Contraindications
* Patients with hypersensitivity to psuedoephedrine or tripolidine
* Should not be given to patients with hypertension, acute asthma, peptic ulcer disease, severe coronary artery disease, arrhythmias, glaucoma, angina pectoris, severe cardiovascular disease or patients taking MAO (monoamine oxidase) inhibitors.
(iii) Side effects
* Can cause drowsiness, dizziness, dry nose, mouth and throat
* May cause restlessness, anxiety, nervousness or insomnia in some patients
* Some patients may experience photosensitivity skin reactions during prolonged sun exposure.
(iv) Dosage-one tablet p.o. (by mouth) every 8 hours
(v) Considerations
* Should be taken with food or milk to reduce gastrointestinal distress
* Patient should avoid alcohol, driving and other activities that require alertness until the CNS effects are known by the patient
* Dry mouth can be relieved with gum, hard candy or ice chips
* Advise patients to use sunblock for possible photosensitivity.
(vi) Common brand name: Actifed

(b) Pseudoephedrine HCL (decongestant)
(i) Indications-Symptomatic relief of nasal congestion associated with rhinitis and sinusitis and for eustachian tube congestion
(ii) Contraindications
* Hypersensitivity to Sudafed
* Severe hypertension
* Coronary artery disease
* Glaucoma
* Hyperthyroidism or for patients taking MAO inhibitors.
(iii) Side effects
* Transient restlessness
* Stimulation
* Tachycardia
* Nervousness
* Dizziness
* Dry mouth.
(iv) Dosage
* 30 - 60 mg P.O. every 4-6 hours for adults

        *   Maximum daily dose (24 hours) is 240 mg.
- (v) Considerations
  - * Drug may act as a stimulant
  - * Avoid taking within 2 hours of bedtime
  - * Advise patient to stop taking medication if extreme restlessness occurs and consult MD/PA
  - * Advise patients that many over the counter (OTC) drugs may contain ephedrine or other sympathomimetic amines and might intensify the action of psuedoephedrine if taken together.
- (vi) Common brand name: Sudafed

- (c) Chlorpheniramine -antihistamine
  - (i) Indications-Symptomatic relief of rhinitis and seasonal allergy symptoms
  - (ii) Contraindications
    - * Hypersensitivity to antihistamines
    - * Lower respiratory tract symptoms
    - * Narrow-angle glaucoma
    - * Severe hypertension
    - * Severe cardiovascular disease
    - * Bronchial asthma
    - * Patients taking MAO inhibitors.
  - (iii) Side effects-Low incidence of side effects
    - * Drowsiness
    - * Dizziness
    - * Dryness of mouth and nose
  - (iv) Dosage
    - * 8 mg P.O. every 8 hours (t.i.d.)
    - * Maximum daily (24 hours) dose is 24 mg.
  - (v) Considerations
    - * Drug may cause drowsiness
    - * Driving and other potentially hazardous activities should be avoided until the response to the drug is known
    - * Avoid alcohol use when taking this drug. Antihistamines have additive effects with alcohol.
  - (vi) Common brand name: Chlor-Trimeton, CTM

- (d) Robitussin (guiafenesin)
  - (i) Indications
    - * Used to liquefy thick tenacious sputum
    - * Expectorant
  - (ii) Contraindications-Contraindicated in patients with known hypersensitivity to the drug
  - (iii) Side effects-rare
    - * GI upset

        *   Nausea
        *   Drowsiness
  (iv) Dosage
        *   200-400 mg P.O. every 4 hours
        *   Maximum daily (24 hours) dose is 2,400 mg.
  (v) Considerations
        *   Take medication with plenty of fluids to help
            liquefy secretions
        *   Persistent cough may indicate a more serious
            problem. Notify MD/PA if cough lasts longer
            than one week
  (vi) Common brand name: Hytuss, Robitussin,
        Humabid

(e) Robitussin DM (Guaifenesin with Dextromethorphan)
    Antitussive/Expectorant
  (i) Indications-Temporary relief of cough spasms in
       nonproductive coughs due to colds and flu
  (ii) Contraindications
        *   Hypersensitivity to the drug
        *   Patients who have asthma
        *   Persistent or chronic coughs or in patients
            taking MAO inhibitors.
  (iii) Side effects-Rare
        *   Dizziness
        *   Drowsiness
        *   Excitability, especially in children
        *   GI upset
        *   Constipation and abdominal discomfort.
  (iv) Dosage
        *   10-20 mg P.O. every 4 hours or 30 mg P.O.
            every 6-8 hours.
        *   Maximum daily (24 hours) dose is 120 mg.
  (v) Considerations
        *   Drug produces no analgesia or addiction and
            little or no CNS depression
        *   Dextromethorphan 15-30 mg is equivalent to
            8-15 mg codeine as an antitussive
        *   Patient should understand that a persistent
            cough might indicate a more serious
            problems
        *   Coughs lasting for longer than a week should
            be evaluated by a MD/PA.
  (vi) Common brand names
        *   Robitussin DM

(f) Diphenhydramine (antihistamine)
  (i) Indications

         *   Temporary symptomatic relief of various allergic conditions and to treat or prevent motion sickness and vertigo
         *   Used in anaphylaxis as an adjunct to epinephrine
         *   Used as a sedative

(ii) Contraindications
         *   Contraindicated in patients who have a known hypersensitivity to the drug
         *   Do not give if patient has acute asthma or an enlarged prostrate gland

(iii) Side Effects
         *   Drowsiness
         *   Dry mouth
         *   Palpitations
         *   Some patients may experience nervousness, restlessness and insomnia.

(iv) Dosage
         *   25 to 50 mg P.O. three times a day (t.i.d.) or four times a day (q.i.d.)
         *   Maximum daily dose (24 hours) is 300 mg.

(v) Considerations
         *   May cause GI upset
         *   Administer with food or milk
         *   Warn patients about possible additive CNS depressant effects with concurrent use of alcohol
         *   Patient should not engage in activities that require alertness and coordination until response to the drug is known
         *   Drowsiness is most prominent during the first few days of therapy and often disappears with continued therapy
         *   The drug has an atropine-like drying effect, which makes it a popular drug for use with the common cold
         *   Antihistamines have no therapeutic effects on the common cold and may make expectoration more difficult because it thickens bronchial secretions
         *   Increase fluid intake while taking this drug.

(vi) Common brand name: Benadryl

Emetics

(a) Syrup of Ipecac

(i) Indications-To induce vomiting in poisoning or overdose by ingestion in a conscious patient

(ii) Contraindications
         *   Stupor or coma
         *   Absent gag reflex

* Seizures
* Pregnancy
* Children under 6, or if the following is ingested: corrosives, hydrocarbons, strychnine or iodides
(iii) Side effects
* The risk of aspiration from vomiting is present.
* If the drug is not vomited, it may cause GI upset, diarrhea or slight CNS depression
* May cause persistent vomiting. Syrup of ipecac can be cardiotoxic if not vomited
(iv) Dosage - only given under orders of MD/PA
* Children 3-5 teaspoons, Adults 1-2 tablespoons P.O.
* Follow administration of the drug with 1-2 glasses of tepid water. Do not give milk products
* May repeat the dose in 20 minutes if no results
(v) Considerations
* Drug should be recovered by gastric lavage and activated charcoal if vomiting does not occur following the second dose
* Notify MD/PA immediately if vomiting does not occur. If poisoning has occurred, call a poison control center or emergency room or contact an MD/PA before using ipecac syrup
* Do not exceed the recommended dosage.
(vi) Common brand name: Syrup of Ipecac

Antidiarrheal
(a) Kaopectate Tabs
(i) Indications-Acute nonspecific diarrhea
(ii) Contraindications - Patients with known hypersensitivity to the drug and in patients with dysentery or suspected bowel obstruction
(iii) Side effects-constipation
(iv) Dosage
* 1.2 to 1.5 grams P.O. after each loose bowel movement
* Not to exceed 9 grams in 24 hours
(v) Considerations
* Use cautiously in patients with dehydration
* Encourage adequate fluid intake to compensate for fluid loss from diarrhea
* Do not use if diarrhea is accompanied by fever or blood or mucous in the stool.
(vi) Common brand names: Kaopectate, Donnagel

(b) Immodium
    (i) Indications-Acute nonspecific diarrhea
    (ii) Side effects-constipation
    (iii) Dosage
        * 2 - 2mg tabs, followed by 1 tab after each
          loose stool
        * Not to exceed 8 tablets a day
        * Do NOT give for bloody diarrhea

Antacids

(a) Calcium Carbonate Tabs
    (i) Indications
        * Used for relief of transient symptoms of
          hyperacidity as in acid indigestion and
          heartburn
        * Also used as a calcium supplement.
    (ii) Contraindications
        * Patients with hypercalcemia and
          hypercalciuria
        * Should also not be used in patients with
          calcium loss due to immobilization, severe
          renal disease, renal calculi, and GI
          hemorrhage or obstruction or cardiac
          disease.
    (iii) Side effects
        * Constipation or laxative effect
        * Acid rebound
        * Nausea
        * Flatulence.
    (iv) Dosage
        * 0.5-2 grams P.O. 4-6 times/day when used
          as an antacid
        * For use as calcium supplement 1-2 grams
          P.O. every 8 or every 12 hours
    (v) Considerations
        * When used as an antacid, take one hour after
          meals and at bedtime
        * Acid rebound, which generally occurs after
          repeated use of antacids for one or two
          weeks, can lead to chronic use
        * Caution patient not to use antacids for more
          than two weeks without medical supervision
    (vi) Common brand names: Tums, Caltrate, Os-Cal

Injectable medications

For pain
(a) Morphine (analgesic, narcotic (opiate) agonist)
    (i) Indications

* Symptomatic relief of severe acute pain after nonnarcotic analgesics has failed
* Also used to relieve pulmonary edema and the pain of myocardial infarction

(ii) Contraindications
* Patients with known hypersensitivity to the drug or to opiates
* Patients with increased intracranial pressure(head injuries), severe respiratory depression, acute bronchial asthma, convulsive disorders, chronic pulmonary diseases and undiagnosed acute abdominal conditions

(iii) Side effects
* Drowsiness
* Pruritus (itching)
* Respiratory depression
* Euphoria
* Disorientation
* Nausea
* Vomiting
* Constipation
* Occasionally patients will experience nervousness, restlessness, or insomnia
* Urinary retention may occur

(iv) Dosage
* 2.5-15 mg intravenous (IV) every 4 hours
* 1 –2 mg IV doses titrated to pain relief
* May also be given intramuscularly (IM) or P.O. (by mouth). IM dosage is 5-20 mg IM every 4 hours
* Oral dosage is 10-30 mg every 4 hours

(v) Considerations
* Monitor for respiratory depression
* Evaluate patient frequently for pain relief
* Patients who are ambulatory may experience nausea and orthostatic hypotension when moving from a supine to an upright position.
* Note: Morphine sulfate is a Schedule II Controlled Substance

(vi) Common brand name: Duramorph, MS Contin(oral)

For chemical agent poisoning
(a) Atropine INJ 0.7 ml
(i) Indications- used to treat a chemical agent poisoning
(ii) Contraindications-None when used for life threatening emergencies
(iii) Side effects

46

* Blurred vision
* Headache
* Pupillary dilatation
* Dry mouth
* Thirst
* Flushing of the skin
* Difficulty in urination

(iv) Dosage-0.5 to 1.0 mg

(b) Diazepam –Anticonvulsant (CANA)
  (i) Indications
  * Used to treat status epilepticus
  * Used for short term relief of anxiety symptoms, to allay anxiety and tension prior to surgery, dental procedures and endoscopic procedures
  * Used alleviate acute withdrawal symptoms of alcoholism

  (vii) Contraindications
  * Patients with known hypersensitivity to the drug
  * Should not be given to patients in profound shock, coma, acute alcohol intoxication, or with depressed vital signs

  (viii) Side effects
  * Drowsiness and sedation
  * Possible hypotension
  * Depressed level of consciousness
  * Some patients may become restless or agitated after administration of the drug.

  (ix) Dosage
  * For seizures/status epilepticus-5 to 10 mg IV (preferred), or IM if IV route not available
  * May repeat every 10-15 minutes as needed up to a maximum of 30 mg
  * For anxiety, the oral route is preferred and the dose is 2-10 mg P.O. anywhere from 2- 4 times a day depending on response.

  (x) Considerations
  * Don't mix diazepam with other drugs and don't store in plastic syringes
  * IV route is the most reliable parenteral route
  * IM administration is not recommended because absorption is variable and injection is painful
  * Give IV not to exceed 5 mg a minute. Avoid the use of small veins, as this drug is very irritating and can cause phlebitis.

  (xi) Common brand name: Valium

(c) Ativan (Lorazepam)
   (i) Indications
      * Anxiety disturbances or anxiety states: general anxiety disturbances panic disturbances phobic anxiety disturbances
      * Adjustment disturbances with anxiety or stress reaction
   (ii) Contraindications
      * Assess patient periodically
      * Safety and efficacy in children under the age of 12 has not been established
   (iii) Dosages
      * ADULT dose for anxiety is: 2mg - 3mg daily in 3 - 4 divided doses
      * RANGE: 1mg - 6mg daily in divided doses
      * ELDERLY/DEBILITATED PATIENTS: Initial dose of 1mg - 2mg/day in divided doses. Adjust as needed and tolerated.
      * In elderly and/or debilitated patients and in those with serious respiratory or cardiovascular disease, a reduction in dosage is recommended
      * In the case of local anaesthesia and diagnostic procedures requiring patient co-operation, concomitant use of an analgesic is recommended.
      * Ativan sl: Dosage of ativan sublingual should be individualized for maximum effect.
   (iv) Pre medication
      * The night before the procedure: The recommended dose is 1 - 2 mg
      * Pre-procedure: The recommended average adult dose is 2mg administered 1 - 2 hours before the procedure
      * If a heightened sedative effect is desired, a dose of 0.05mg/kg to a maximum of 4mg may be used

(d) 2-PAM Cl
   (i) Indications
      * Relieves the symptom of skeletal neuromuscular blockade
      * Simultaneous administration of atropine is required
   (ii) Contraindications
      * Can produce drowsiness, headache, disturbance of vision, nausea, dizzziness, tachycardi and anincrase in blood pressure, hyperventilation and muscular weakness

For anaphylaxis
(a) Epinephrine 1:1000(1 mg/1cc) -bronchodilator

(i)   Indications-Used for bronchospasm, hypersensitivity (allergic) reactions and anaphylaxis

(ii) Contraindications
* Patients with known hypersensitivity to the drug
* Patients with narrow-angle glaucoma, hemorrhagic, traumatic or cardiogenic shock, cardiac arrhythmias or coronary insufficiency.

(iii) Side effects
* Nervousness
* Restlessness
* Palpitations
* Tremors
* Fear
* Anxiety
* Headache
* Hypertension
* Nausea and vomiting

(iv) Dosage-0.1-0.5cc SC (subcutaneous) every 15 minutes as needed to treat acute symptoms

(v) Considerations
* Drug of choice for acute anaphylactic reactions
* Patients allergic to insect stings should be taught to self administer epinephrine
* Closely monitor vital signs after administration of the drug.

(vi) Common brand names: Adrenalin Chloride, Epi-Pen

Topical medications

(a) Bacitracin Ointment-Local Anti-infective

(i)   Indications-Used topically in the treatment of superficial infections of the skin.

(ii) Contraindications
* Contraindicated in patients with known hypersensitivity to the drug
* Patients allergic to neomycin may also be allergic to bacitracin

(iii) Side effects
* Itching and burning have also been reported with topical use.

(iv) Dosage-Apply a thin layer of ointment twice a day or three times a day.

(v) Consideration
* Watch for signs of local allergic manifestations such as redness, itching and burning
* Clean skin before applying the drug

(vi) Common brand names: Bacitracin

(b) Hydrocortisone 1% cream-topical anti-inflammatory
    (i) Indications-For relief of inflammation and pruritus associated contact dermatitis
    (ii) Contraindications-Patients with known hypersensitivity to the drug or its components
    (iii) Side effects
       * Maceration of the skin
       * Secondary infection
    (iv) Dosage - Apply ointment to affected area sparingly daily to four times a day until acute phase is controlled, then reduce dosage to one to three times weekly, as needed.
    (v) Considerations
       * Gently wash skin before applying ointment
       * Avoid applying near eyes or mucous membranes
       * May be safely used on the face, groin, armpits and under breasts.
    (vi) Common brand names
       * Cortizone-5
       * Bactine Hydrocortisone
       * Acticort 100

(c) Miconozole 2% cream-anti-fungal
    (i) Indications-Used to treat tinea pedis (athlete's foot), tinea cruris and tinea corporis
    (ii) Contraindications-Contraindicated in patients with known hypersensitivity to the drug.
    (iii) Side effects
       * Skin irritation
       * Burning
       * Maceration
       * Allergic contact dermatitis.
    (iv) Dosage-Apply sparingly twice a day to the affected area for 2-4 weeks.
    (v) Considerations
       * Instruct patient how to cleanse area prior to application of cream
       * Apply sparingly in skin-fold areas and massage in well to prevent maceration.
    (vi) Common brand names: Micatin

(d) Clortrimozole Cream- Anti-fungal
    (i) Indications-Used to treat dermal fungal infections, tinea pedis, tinea cruris and tinea corporis
    (ii) Contraindications-Patients with known hypersensitivity to the drug or its components
    (iii) Side effects

        * Stinging
        * Erythema
        * Edema vesication
        * Pruritis and urticaria

(iv) Dosage-Apply small amount to affected area twice a day, A.M. and P.M., or as directed by the physician.

(v) Considerations
* Apply to dry skin
* Cleanse skin thoroughly before applying the medication
* Signs of clinical improvement should be anticipated within one week of use. Report signs of condition worsening, skin irritation or no improvement after 4 weeks of therapy

(vi) Common brand names: Lotrimin, Mycelex

(e) Dibucaine Ointment-local anesthetic

(i) Indications-Used for temporary relief of pain and itching due to hemorrhoids and other anorectal disorders, nonpoisonous insect bites, sunburn, minor burns, cuts and scratches.

(ii) Contraindications-Patients with known hypersensitivity to the drug or its components.

(iii) Side effects
* Skin irritation
* Contact dermatitis
* Rectal bleeding (suppository use)

(iv) Dosage
* Apply skin cream or ointment to affected areas, as needed (max 1 oz in 24 hours)
* Insert rectal ointment morning and evening and after each bowel movement.

(v) Considerations
* The cream preparation is water soluble and therefore should be applied after bathing or swimming
* Caution patient to use medication only as directed
* Medication is intended only for temporary relief of mild to moderate itching or pain

(vi) Common brand names: Nupercainal

Antibiotics

Penicillin

(a) Indications

(i) Penicillin administered intravenously is a primary drug of choice for bacterial meningitis if this disease is caused by sensitive strains of

meningococci or pneumococci. Further important indications for an intravenous penicillin treatment are an endocarditis caused by streptococcus viridans, other streptococcal infections (severe pneumonia, arthiritis), neurosyphilis, actinomycosis, anthrax, and clostridium infections.
(ii) Smaller doses are administered intramuscularly. A streptococcal pharyngitis can be treated with a single injection of a benzylpenicillin slow release preparation (if available). Erysipelas, diphtheria, pneumococcal pneumonia, and primary syphilis infections can also be treated intramuscularly. Secondary prophylaxis of rheumatic fever has become very rare.
(iii) Orally administered Penicillin VK is a "painless" alternative for streptoccal infections. It can be considered in the early stages of Lyme disease if doxycycline is contraindicated.
(b) Contraindications: None except hypersensitivity to penicillin
(c) Cautions: If a meningococcal infection is suspected, parenteral penicillin therapy ought to be started as quickly as possible.
(d) Adverse Reactions
(i) Severe penicillin hypersensitivity with anaphylactic shock is very rare and occurs mostly in connexion with parenteral administration (5 to 10 cases on 10000 treated subjects). The emergency treatment is based primarily on epinephrine (and, in addition, maybe intravenous corticosteroids).
(ii) Hypersensitive skin reactions (skin rashes, urticaria) are frequent (1 to 7% of the treated subjects). A sterile abscess can occur at the area of the i.m. injection. Hemolytic anemia, nephritis, and liver granuloma are very rare complications. Massive i.v. doses are associated to a risk of an electrolyte and volume overload.
(iii) Oral preparations occasionally cause nausea, vomiting, or diarrhea.
(e) Risk groups
(i) Pregnant women: Can be given. Penicillin is considered the safest antibiotic during pregnancy.
(ii) Nursing mothers: Can be given. Concentrations in breast milk are relatively low. The risk of an alteration of the child's intestinal flora or of a hypersensitivation cannot be excluded.
(iii) Children: Intravenously for severe infections: 0.2 to 0.5 million I.U./kg/day in 4 to 6 doses. Oral (penicillin V): 100,000 I.U./kg/day in two doses (a maximum of 1.5 million I.U./day).

    (iv) Elderly people: No dose reduction is necessary if renal functions are normal.

    (v) Renal failure: Creatinine clearance less than 50 ml/min: reduce dose by 25 to 50%; clearance less than 10 ml/min: reduce dose by 50-75%.

    (vi) Liver insufficiency: No dose adjustment necessary

Doxycycline (Oral)

(a) Indications

    (i) Doxycycline is effective for selected infections of the upper respiratory tract or of the (genito-) urinary tract

    (ii) Particularly well suited for atypical pneumonia (as long as a legionella infection can be excluded), for disease following chlamydia trachomatis (non-gonorrheal urethritis, acute urethral syndrome, venereal lymphogranuloma, etc.), for rickettsial diseases (Rocky Mountatin spotted fever, Q fever), for cholera, and for anthrax. Doxycycline can be applied in stage I of Lyme disease. The efficacy for papulopustular acne is also well documented.

    (iii) Doxycycline is considered an alternative drug for syphilis when there is e.g. a hypersensitivity to penicillin.

    (iv) Recommended as a follow-up treatment to a single dose of ceftriaxone for the treatment of possible chlamydia infections in context with gonorrhea

    (v) Used in combination with other antibiotics for acute adnexites caused by mixed infections

    (vi) Used for the prophylaxis of traveler's diarrhea

    (vii) Also considered for the prevention or treatment of multiresistant malaria (e.g. in Thailand)

(b) Contraindications

    (i) Pregnant women: Disturbances in the development of the teeth and bones of the fetus. Can be hepatotoxic for the mother in isolated cases.

    (ii) Nursing mothers: Most specialists allow breast-feeding: it appears only in small amounts in breast milk; risks for child and mother are probably minimal.

    (iii) Children: Contraindicated before the age of eight! (Staining of the teeth and possibly disturbed bone growth.) Older children: 2 to 4 mg/kg/day, may be divided into two doses.

    (iv) Renal failure: Some authors recommend a dose reduction when there is severe insufficiency

(c) Adverse Reactions

(i) Approximately 3 to 4% of the treated subjects complain about nausea
(ii) Abdominal pains and diarrhea are less common
(iii) Esophageal ulcerations have been observed after the administration of doxycycline capsules (do not take before retiring to bed!)
(iv) Like other tetracyclines, doxycycline can lead to staining of the teeth and bone problems in the developing age. Allergic skin reactions occur in about 2%
(v) Doxycycline can cause a cutaneous photosensitivity - inform patient increase risk of sunburn, sensitive to sun and to wear sunscreen
(d) Interactions
(i) Concomitant administration of antacids, calcium-, magnesium-, and iron-salts has a chelating effect and therefore causes a reduced absorption of the antibiotic
(e) Caution: Doxycycline can also be injected intravenously

Cefazolin (Injection)
(a) Indications
(i) Respiratory infections caused by S.pneumoniae, Klebsiella, H.influenzae S.aureus, group A beta-haemolytic streptococci
(ii) Genito-urinary infections caused by E.coli, P.mirabilis, Klebsiella, some strains of enterococci and Enterobacter
(iii) Skin and soft tissue infections due to S.aureus, and group A beta- haemolytic streptococci and other strains of streptococci
(iv) Biliary tract infections due to E.coli and Klebsiella species
(v) Bone and joint infections due to S.aureus.
(vi) Septicaemia due to S.pneumoniae, S.aureus, P.mirabilis, E.coli and Klebsiella species
(vii) Endocarditis due to S.aureus and group A beta-haemolytic streptococci. Appropriate culture and susceptibility studies should be performed to determine susceptibility of the causative organism to cefazolin.
(viii) Peri-operative prophylaxis: Cefazolin is useful in pre-operative, intra-operative and post-operative prophylaxis in various surgical procedures.This is especially effective in reducing the post-operative infections due to contaminated or potentially contaminated surgical procedures. The preoperative use of cefazolin may also be effective in surgical patients in whom infection at the operative site would present a serious risk. The prophylactic administration of cefazolin should

usually be discontinued within a 24-hour period after surgical procedure. NOTE: Susceptibility studies should be performed.

    (ix) Bacteriology
-     Staphylococcus Aureus (penicillin sensitive and resistant)
-     Group A beta-haemolytic streptococci and other strains of streptococci (many strains of enterococci are resistant)
-     Escherichia coli
-     Proteus mirabilis
-     Klebsiella species
-     Enterobacter aerogenes
-     Haemophilus influenzae

(b) Contra-Indications
- (i) Cross sensitivity to Penicillin. About 10% of people allergic to penicillin will also be allergic to Cefozolin
- (ii) Hypersensitivity to cephalosporins
- (iii) Safety in pregnancy, lactation and infants under one month of age has not been established and as such is not recommended

(c) Dosage: Management of overdose
- (i) Rx: Symptomatic and supportive

(d) Side-Effects
- (i) Drug fever
- (ii) Skin rash
- (iii) Vulvar pruritis
- (iv) Nausea
- (v) Vomiting
- (vi) Anorexia
- (vii) Diarrhea
- (ix) Genital and anal pruritis
- (x) Genital moniliasis and vaginitis
- (xi) Phlebitis at the site of injection and after I/M administration, pain at site of injection

(e) Precautions:
- (i) Allergic reaction warrants immediate withdrawal of the drug with appropriate treatment.
- (ii) Caution in patients with penicillin sensitivities as cross sensitivity has been noted.
- (iii) Prolonged use may cause overgrowth of non-susceptible organisms.
- (iv) Caution in patients with low urinary output because of impaired renal function. A lower daily dose is required.
- (v) Pseudomembranous colitis has been reported with broad spectrum antibiotics including cefazolin, therefore it is important to consider it's diagnosis in patients who develop diarrhea in association with

it's use. Such colitis may be life threatening and appropriate measure should be taken, including discontinuation of the anti-biotic

(vi) Pregnancy:
* Safety in pregnancy, lactation, premature infants and infants under one month has not been established.
* Many cephalosporins have been used in pregnancy without any apparent ill effect to the mother or fetus.

(f) Brand Name
(i) Ancef®
(ii) Kefzol

Clinical Handbook

Supportive Care 4

This page intentionally left blank.

91W10
Advanced Individual
Training Course

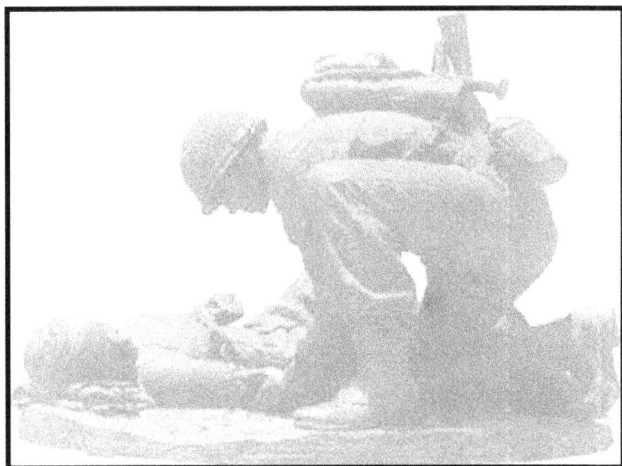

Clinical Handbook
Supportive Care 4

Department of the Army
Academy of Health Sciences
Fort Sam Houston, Texas 78234

Appendix A – Wound Care, Competency Skill Sheets

Appendix B - Cardiac Monitoring, Competency Skill Sheets

Appendix C –Respiratory Care, Competency Skill Sheets

i

TERMINAL LEARNING OBJECTIVE
Given a deceased casualty provide post-mortem care.

Process Used to Declare a Person Dead
Hospital policies state who is responsible for pronouncing the death of the patient. The physician is the best qualified and is usually responsible for declaring a person dead.

Changes That Occur in the Body after Death
Post-mortem Cooling (Algor Mortis)
(1)   Occurs when no further heat is produced by metabolism. Body temperature falls gradually after death (approximately 1.0 to 1.5 degrees F/hr.)

(2)   Cooling continues until room temperature is reached in about 24 hours

Muscular Rigidity (Rigor Mortis)
(1)   Begins about 6 hours after death

(2)   First evident in the muscles of the jaw, then extends to involve all the muscles in the body 12 to 14 hours after death

(3)   Condition where the muscles become rigid. The body is fixed in the position in which it lies.

Purple Discoloration (Livor Mortis)
(1)   Reddish-purple discoloration that develops in the dependent parts of a dead body

(2)   First evident about 30 minutes after death and fully developed in 6-10 hours

(3)   Discoloration is caused by blood flowing passively into the dependent parts of the body

Decomposition (Putrefaction)
(1)   The destruction of a dead body by bacteria

(2)   The rate at which changes develop depends on the environment. Hot, moist conditions favor putrefaction, but cold, dry air delays or prevent it.

(3)   The body of the deceased should be placed in refrigeration in the morgue as soon as possible

(4)   It is best not to keep the body on the nursing unit more than one hour

(5)   Embalming is used as a method of chemically preserving the body. A solution is introduced into the body that kills the bacteria and prevents the rapid decomposition of tissues.

Death Certificate
U.S. laws require that a death certificate be prepared for each person who dies.

Death certificates are sent to local health departments, which compile statistics from the information

A physician is usually responsible for declaring a person dead and is required to sign the death certificate

Organ Donation and Autopsy
Patients who express a wish to donate functional organs after death should be provided an organ donor consent card

The family of a deceased client may decide to donate the client's organs and should also be provided with information and consent forms

An autopsy is an examination of the organs and tissue of a human body after death

The closest surviving family member usually has the authority to consent for an autopsy
(1)   It is usually the physician's responsibility to obtain permission for an autopsy
(2)   The client may have granted permission before his death
(3)   If the death was caused by accident, suicide, homicide, or illegal therapeutic practice, the coroner must be notified and he will decide if an autopsy is necessary
(4)   The family's consent is not needed in these cases
(5)   Many relatives find comfort when they are told that the knowledge gained from an autopsy may contribute to advancements in medical science as well as establish the exact cause of death

Responsibility in Preparing the Body
a.   Provide privacy for the patient and/or family
b.   Verify that the patient has died, and has been pronounced dead by the physician
c.   Notify appropriate persons in the hospital, as well as the clergy, if requested by the family
d.   Obtain the death pack
e.   Wear gloves when preparing the body
f.   Position the body supine in proper alignment, close the eyelids, and place a pillow under the head. If the eyes are to be donated, place a small ice pack on each eye.
g.   Change all dressings; if appropriate, remove jewelry and eyeglasses and place with personal belongings, and replace dentures, if possible
h.   Bathe the body
(1)   Using plain water, wash the areas of the body that may be soiled with blood, feces, or emesis
(2)   If drainage occurs around the rectum, urethra or vagina, place a gauze 4 X 4 over each opening and secure it with tape to prevent further soiling
i.   Arrange the hair neatly
j.   Care of drainage and other tubes
(1)   If there is to be an autopsy, the tubes are generally left in the body
(2)   Remove the drainage bottles or bags from the tubes and fold the tubes over twice; secure each with a rubber band to avoid leakage

       (3)   Make sure you deflate the balloon tips so as not to injure the body tissues upon removal

k.   Apply a clean patient gown and clean bed linen if the family will be viewing the body; leave the head uncovered and have the room arranged neatly

l.   Prepare the family before viewing the body: offer support and your physical presence if desired, during their visit, and assist them with funeral arrangements, if necessary

m.   Identify and assemble the patient's personal belongings for the family; complete a full inventory of the patient's belongings

n.   Attach 3 forms of identification. Two tags are placed on the body (usually the great toe and the wrist). A third tag is placed on the shroud or zippered bag.

o.   You may need to tie a bandage lightly under the jaw and up around the head to keep the jaw closed

p.   Lightly bandage the wrists together, criss- crossed over the abdomen to prevent the arms from falling off the stretcher when the body is being moved to the morgue

q.   Place the body within the shroud or zippered bag

r.   Transport the body to the morgue
       (1)   Place the body on a stretcher and secure it with straps

s.   Record the procedure before the body leaves the nursing unit
       (1)   Record the time and date body was taken to the morgue or by the undertaker
       (2)   If valuables were placed in safekeeping, indicate this in writing
       (3)   If valuables were given to the family or friends, record name of the person(s) to whom they were given, their relationship to the deceased, and the time and date
       (4)   Have a co-worker who witnessed this action co-sign with you in the notes

Role in Caring for the Family of the Deceased Client
    After death, the soldier medic must continue to provide care for the family of the deceased client
       (1)   Listen to the family's expression of grief and loss
       (2)   Allow family members to see the client's body. This will help them to accept the death fully.
       (3)   Provide a private place for the family to grieve and make necessary arrangements
       (4)   Contact the chaplain if the family requests

Deaths on the Battlefield
- On the battlefield when KIA's are identified a spot report is generated identifying the location of the remains so that when the battle is over the remains can be recovered and turned over to mortuary affairs.

- It is standard to use a 10 digit grid coordinate
       (1)   10 Digit Grid coordinate will identify a 1 square meter location within a grid square for the location of the body
       (2)   A global positioning system (GPS) can also be used to document the location of a body

TERMINAL LEARNING OBJECTIVE
Given a standard fully stocked Combat Medic Vest System (CMVS) or fully stocked M5 Bag, you encounter a casualty with an open wound who is breathing. The casualty has been initially assessed and injury(ies) prioritized.

Closed wound injury
(1) Contusion - Hematoma beneath unbroken skin because of small vessel ruptures
(2) Crush injuries - Overlying skin may remain intact, injury to multiple tissues, muscle or bone injury

Open wound injury
(1) Abrasions - Partial thickness skin loss
(2) Lacerations - Break in skin of varying depth
(3) Avulsion - Full thickness skin loss, degloving or flap injuries are avulsions
(4) Amputations - A part of the body is partially or completely severed or torn from the body
(5) Punctures/ penetrations - Caused by a foreign object that enters the body, underlying damage can be extensive
(6) Bite - Breakage of the skin caused by animal or human teeth, all bites are considered contaminated

Identify forms of wound healing
Three types of wound healing
(1) Primary intention (primary union)
  (a) Wounds that are made surgically
  (b) Little tissue loss
  (c) Skin edges are close together and minimal scarring
  (d) Healing begins during the inflammatory phase
(2) Secondary intention (granulation)
  (a) Healing occurs when skin edges are not close together (approximated) or when pus has formed
  (b) If wound is producing or containing pus (purulent) a drainage system is established or the wound is packed with gauze
  (c) Slowly the necrotized tissue decomposes and escapes
  (d) The cavity begins to fill with soft, pink, fleshy projections consisting of capillaries surrounded by fibrous collagen (granulation tissue)
  (e) The amount of granulation tissue required depends on the size of the wound
  (f) Scarring is greater in a large wound
(3) Tertiary (third) intention
  (a) Delayed primary closer
  (b) Two layers of granulation tissue are sutured together
  (c) Occurs when:
    (i) Contaminated wound is left open and sutured closed after the infection is controlled
    (ii) Delayed suturing of a wound

(iii)   Primary wound becomes infected, is opened, is allowed to granulate, and is then sutured

(d)   Results in a larger and deeper scar than primary or secondary intention

Factors promoting wound healing

(1)   Adequate oxygenation

(2)   Adequate rest or local immobilization

(3)   Sufficient blood supply

(4)   Proper nutrition

    (a)   Nutrients are needed for wound repair and prevention of infection

    (b)   Adequate wound healing is dependent upon the availability of essential nutrients

Factors that impair wound healing

(1)   Age - causes slower regeneration of tissue

    (a)   Physiological Effects

        (i)   Alters all phases of wound healing

        (ii)   Vascular changes impair circulation to wound site

        (iii)   Reduced liver function alters synthesis of clotting factors

        (iv)   Formation of antibodies and lymphocytes is reduced

        (v)   Collagen tissue is less pliable

        (vi)   Scar tissue is less elastic

    (b)   Interventions

        (i)   Instruct patient on safety precautions to avoid injuries

        (ii)   Be prepared to provide wound care for longer period

        (iii)   Teach home caregivers wound care techniques

(2)   Malnutrition

    (a)   Physiological Effects

        (i)   All phases of wound healing are impaired

        (ii)   Stress from burns or severe trauma increases nutritional requirements

    (b)   Interventions

        (i)   Provide balanced diet rich in protein, carbohydrates, lipids, vitamins A and C, and minerals

(3)   Obesity

    (a)   Physiological Effects

        (i)   Fatty tissue lacks adequate blood supply to resist bacterial infection and deliver nutrients and cellular elements

    (b)   Interventions

        (i)   Observe obese patient for signs of wound infection, dehiscence, and evisceration

(4)   Impaired oxygenation
- (a) Physiological Effects
  - (i) Low arterial oxygen tension alters synthesis of collagen and formation of epithelial cells
  - (ii) If local circulating blood flow is poor, tissues fail to receive needed oxygen
  - (iii) Decreased hemoglobin (anemia) reduces arterial oxygen levels in capillaries and interferes with tissue repair
- (b) Interventions
  - (i) Diet adequate in iron
  - (ii) Monitor patients' hematocrit and hemoglobin levels

(5)   Smoking
- (a) Physiological Effects
  - (i) Reduces the amount of functional hemoglobin in blood, thus decreasing tissue oxygenation
  - (ii) May increase platelet aggregation and cause hypercoagulability
  - (iii) Interferes with normal cellular mechanisms that promote release of oxygen to tissue
- (b) Interventions
  - (i) Discourage patient from smoking by explaining its effects on wound healing

(6)   Presence of infection

(7)   Drugs
- (a) Physiological Effects
  - (i) Steroids reduce inflammatory response
  - (ii) Anti-inflammatory drugs suppress protein synthesis, wound contraction, epithelialization, and inflammation
  - (iii) Prolonged antibiotic use may increase risk of superinfection
  - (iv) Chemotherapeutic drugs can depress bone marrow function, number of leukocytes, and inflammatory response
- (b) Interventions
  - (i) Carefully observe patient; signs of inflammation may not be obvious

(8)   Chronic diseases that interfere with oxygenation and transport of nutrients
- (a) Physiological Effects

                (i)   Chronic disease causes small blood vessel disease that impairs tissue perfusion

                (ii)   Diabetes causes hemoglobin to have greater affinity for oxygen, so it fails to release oxygen to tissues

                (iii)   Hyperglycemia alters ability of leukocytes to perform phagocytosis and also supports overgrowth of fungal and yeast infection

      (b)   Interventions

                (i)   Instruct patient to take preventive measures to avoid cuts or breaks in skin

                (ii)   Provide preventive foot care

                (iii)   Control blood sugar to reduce the physiological changes associated with diabetes

Assessment considerations

Obtain history of wound injury

(1)   How did the wound occur?

(2)   What type of object caused the injury?

(3)   When did the wound occur?

(4)   Color

      (a)   Pink - usually indicates healthy tissue

      (b)   Black - indicates poor tissue perfusion, necrosis

      (c)   Red - indicates infection

(5)   Odor - a foul smell indicates presence of bacteria

(6)   Wound size –

      (a)   Measure wound from side to side at largest point

      (b)   Take second measurement perpendicular to first

      (c)   Document both measurement (i.e., "1" by "3"), or by using commonly-known object, such as "dime-sized" wound

(7)   Wound boundaries - edges of wound smooth or irregular

(8)   Drainage

      (a)   Color

      (b)   Quantity

      (c)   Consistency (watery, thick, etc.)

      (d)   Odor

Neurovascular status of the affected extremity MUST be assessed prior to wound treatment

(1)   Pulse quality, location, rate

(2)   Capillary refill

(3)   Skin color/temperature

(4)   Sensation/Motor function

Assess the wound

(1)   Contusion

      (a)   Assess for depth of hematoma

      (b)   Identify damage to underlying vessels, nerves and bony structures

	(c)			Assess peripheral pulses
	(d)			Assess sensation
	(e)			Assess motor function and strength
	(f)			Assess for pain control
	(g)			Assess tetanus prophylaxis status

(2) Crush injury
- (a) Assess for wound depth and blood loss
- (b) Assess for neurovascular status:
  - (i) Pulse quality, location, rate
  - (ii) Capillary refill
  - (iii) Skin color
  - (iv) Level of consciousness
- (c) Assess for pain control
- (d) Assess tetanus prophylaxis status

(3) Abrasion
- (a) Assess for amount of fluid loss in large wounds
- (b) Assess functional capabilities
- (c) Assess for pain control
- (d) Assess tetanus prophylaxis status

(4) Laceration
- (a) Assess age and depth
- (b) Assess degree and/or type of contamination
- (c) Assess for associated injuries
- (d) Assess neurovascular status of affected extremity as appropriate:
  - (i) Pulse quality, location, rate
  - (ii) Capillary refill
  - (iii) Skin color/temperature
  - (iv) Sensation/motor function
- (e) Assess for pain control
- (f) Assess tetanus prophylaxis status

(5) Avulsion
- (a) Assess amount of tissue and functional loss
- (b) Assess depth of injury
- (c) Assess for pain control
- (d) Assess for tetanus prophylaxis status

(6) Amputations
- (a) Assess for blood loss and bleeding source
- (b) Assess neurovascular status:
  - (i) Pulse quality, location, rate
  - (ii) Capillary refill
  - (iii) Skin color/temperature
  - (iv) Sensation/motor function
- (c) Assess for pain control
- (d) Assess for tetanus prophylaxis status

(7) Punctures/ penetrations
- (a) Assess for presence of foreign bodies/materials and impaled objects
- (b) Assess depth of penetration for underlying structural damage

(c)   Assess type/degree of contamination
(d)   Assess for pain control
(e)   Assess for tetanus prophylaxis status

Emergency treatment of specific wound types
General treatment
(1)   Life-threatening injuries are managed prior to isolated wounds:
        Assess for and treat any existing critical injuries
        (a)   Airway
        (b)   Breathing
        (c)   Circulation
(2)   Wound categories
        (a)   Penetrating chest wounds
        (b)   Impaled or open abdominal wounds
        (c)   Amputations
        (4)   Avulsions
        (5)   Crush injury
(3)   Expose area
(4)   Stop the bleeding
(5)   Maintain intravenous access and fluids for significant blood loss or
        severe underlying structure damage: Treat for shock as necessary
(6)   Assess for neurovascular status:
        (a)   Pulse quality, location, rate
        (b)   Capillary refill
        (c)   Skin color/temperature
        (d)   Sensation/motor function
(7)   Emergency treatment of specific wounds
        (a)   Cleanse wound to decrease contamination
        (b)   Prevent dehydration of wound by covering wound with
                sterile dressing
(8)   Assess and apply appropriate type of dressing and splints
(9)   Assess activity restrictions
(10)   Provide pain relief management
        (a)   Apply ice packs
        (b)   Administer medication

Specific treatment

(1)   Contusion
        (a)   Elevate contused area or extremity
        (b)   Apply ice pack within first 24 hrs
(2)   Crush injury
        (a)   Control bleeding
                (i)   Direct pressure
                (ii)   Pressure dressing
        (b)   Apply dry, sterile dressing
        (c)   Elevate extremity, if possible
        (d)   Administer antibiotics as directed and tetanus
(3)   Abrasion

  (a) Cleanse wounds thoroughly by scrubbing with normal saline
  (b) Remove debris and foreign bodies with soaked sponge or irrigation
  (c) Apply antibiotic ointment
  (d) Leave wound uncovered or covered with a nonadherent dressing
 (4) Laceration
  (a) Control bleeding with direct pressure
  (b) Cleanse and irrigate thoroughly
  (c) Wound closure by skin sutures, staples or steri-strips
   (i) Sutures - thread, wire or other materials used to sew body tissues together
    * Placed within tissue layers in deep wounds and superficially as the final means for wound closure
    * Deeper sutures are usually made of material that will be absorbed by the body in several days
    * Types: Interrupted or separate, continuous, blanket, retention suture covered with rubber tubing to provide greater strength
   (i) Staples
    * Provides quick closure
    * Usually less costly
    * Limited to areas of less cosmetic importance such as scalp or trunk
    * Removal of staples requires a sterile staple extractor and maintenance of aseptic technique
 (5) Avulsion
  (a) Control bleeding by direct pressure
  (b) Cleanse thoroughly
  (c) Cover wound with ointment, sterile dressing, and splints
 (6) Amputations
  (a) Control bleeding with direct pressure, pressure points and elevation
   (i) Apply tourniquet if above measures are not successful
  (b) Apply moist, sterile dressing over amputation stump
  (c) Wrap amputated body part in moist, sterile dressing; place in plastic bag and place over ice
 (7) Punctures/ penetrations
  (a) Secure any impaled objects
  (b) Soak the wound in warm solution for several minutes
  (c) Provide care of drains, if present
  (d) Administer antibiotics as directed and tetanus

Care for a wound
Types of dressing
   (1)   Gauze dressing
          (a)   Permit air to reach the wound
          (b)   Sterile dressings
   (2)   Semiocclusive dressing
          (a)   Permit oxygen but not air to pass
          (b)   Thought to promote healing by keeping wounds moist (yet sterile) so epithelial cells can slide more easily over the surface of the wound
   (3)   Occlusive dressing
          (a)   Permit neither oxygen or air to pass
          (b)   Thought to promote healing by keeping wounds moist (yet sterile) so epithelial cells can slide more easily over the surface of the wound
          (c)   Tape strips are placed on all sides of the dressing

Changing of dressing
   (1)   Dressings are changed per doctor's orders, when the wound requires assessment or care, and when they become loose or saturated with drainage
   (2)   Supplies and equipment needed
          (a)   Waterproof bed pads
          (b)   Sterile dressings
          (c)   Plastic bag or basin
          (d)   Sterile saline or water
          (e)   Irrigation pack and solution
          (f)   Eye shield or face guard
          (g)   Sterile and clean gloves
          (h)   Tape or Montgomery straps
   (3)   Explain procedure to patient
          (a)   Gather supplies and wash hands
          (b)   Position the patient and expose the area to be redressed
          (c)   Place waterproof pad under patient and prepare plastic bag as receptacle
          (d)   Put on clean non-sterile exam gloves
          (e)   Gently loosen tape toward the wound while supporting the skin around the wound or untie Montgomery straps
          (f)   Remove the dressing, being careful not to tear the wound or dislodge any drains. Use sterile saline to moisten dressing if it is sticking to the wound, to prevent discomfort to the patient and/or to maintain integrity of sutures.
          (g)   Assess amount, color, odor, and consistency of drainage
          (h)   Remove gloves and dispose in plastic bag
          (i)   Establish a sterile field. Open all sterile equipment and supplies and place within the sterile field. Uncap sterile saline or other solution as ordered
          (j)   Put on sterile gloves

Cleansing the wound
    (1)   Linear wound
        (a)   First stroke - cleanse the area directly over the wound by wiping from the top to bottom. Discard the gauze.
        (b)   Second stroke - cleanse the skin area on one side next to the wound, wiping from top to bottom. Discard the gauze.
        (c)   Third stroke - cleanse the skin on other side of wound, wiping from top to bottom. Discard the gauze.
        (d)   Continue this procedure alternating sides of the wound, working away from the wound until clean.
    (2)   Circular wound
        (a)   First stroke - starting at the center of the wound, wipe the wound area with an outward spiral motion. Do not use the same swab/gauze to clean the entire wound
        (b)   Continue this procedure, working outward until wound is clean. Do not cross back to the center of wound.

Irrigate the wound
    (1)   Put on sterile gloves and eye shield or face guard, if available
    (2)   To prevent contamination and to clean the bottle rim, pour a small amount of the liquid into waste receptacle. If the seal of the bottle has not been broken, this step is not necessary
    (3)   Pour irrigating solution into basin with the label facing the palm
    (4)   Fill the syringe with solution from the sterile basin

CAUTION: If Betadine (iodine) is being used, check to ensure patient does not have allergies to the iodine. An alternate, non-iodine-based solution may be used (Hibiclens, phisohex, hydrogen peroxide).

    (5)   Hold the tip of the syringe just above top end of wound and force fluid into the wound slowly and continuously. Use enough force to flush out debris but do not squirt or splash fluid
    (6)   Irrigate all portions of the wound. DO NOT force solution into wound pockets. Continue irrigating until solution draining from bottom end of wound is clear
    (7)   Using sterile gauze, gently pat dry the edges of the wound. Work from cleanest to most contaminated areas

Apply a sterile dressing

    (1)   Lay inner dressing over wound ensuring the dressing extends past the edge of the wound
    (2)   All other dressings will overlap each other and cover entire wound
    (3)   Cover all inner dressings with a large out dressing

CAUTION: Some wounds must be kept moist, and will require the use of "wet to dry" dressings. The inner dressings that touch the wound directly will be dampened with a solution (usually normal saline) before application. The outer dressings are applied dry. Example: abdominal evisceration.

WARNING: During combat conditions, the medic will NOT remove an existing dressing but will only reinforce with additional dressings. Label the dressing "REINFORCED." Write date, time and your initials.

(4)   Remove gloves and place in disposal bag
(5)   Tape the dressing or tie Montgomery straps

CAUTION: Tape should not form a constricting band around the wound or extremity.

(6)   Reposition and cover patient
(7)   Close and dispose of plastic bag with used supplies IAW local policy
(8)   Wash hands
(9)   Document wound care and all assessments on the appropriate form
    (a)   Enter the date and time of the procedure
    (b)   Enter a description of the wound's color, odor, consistency, and amount of drainage

Drainage and drainage systems
Wound drainage
(1)   Exudate –fluid, cells or other substances that have slowly exuded or discharged from cells or blood vessels through small pores or breaks in cell membrane
(2)   Drainage – the removal of fluids from a body cavity, wound, or other source of discharge by one or more methods
(3)   Types
    (a)   Serous
        (i)   Clear, watery fluid that has been separated from its solid elements (e.g., the exudate from a blister)
        (ii)   Serous fluid has characteristics of serum
        (iii)   Serum is clear, thin, sticky fluid portion of blood that remains after coagulation
    (b)   Sanguineous
        (i)   Fluid contains blood
    (c)   Serosanguineous
        (i)   Thin and red, described as pink
(4)   Exudate/drainage greater than 300 ml in the first 24 hours should be treated as abnormal
(5)   When patients first ambulate, a slight increase may occur
(6)   If sanguineous drainage continues, small blood vessels may be oozing
(7)   Not all surgical wounds drain, the following characteristics are important to note and chart:
    (a)   Color
    (b)   Amount
    (c)   Consistency (thick/thin)
    (d)   Odor

Wound drainage systems
(1)   Open drainage
    (a)   Drainage that passes through an open-ended tube into a receptacle or out onto the dressing

(b) Penrose drain is a soft tube that may be „advanced" or pulled out in stages as the wound heals from the inside out

(2) Closed / Suction drainage
 (a) Self-contained suction units that connects to drainage tubes within the wound
 (b) Removes fluid in an airtight circuit
 (c) Prevents environmental contaminates from entering the wound or cavity
 (d) Two types of drainage devices that are portable and provide constant low-pressure suction to remove and collect drainage without wall suction
 (i) Jackson-Pratt drain – used when small amounts (100 –200 ml) of drainage is anticipated
 (ii) Hemovac drainage system used for larger amounts (up to 500 ml) of drainage

Assist with on-going casualty management
Evaluation of wound healing
(1) Checked after:
 (a) Each dressing change
 (b) Application of heat and cold therapies
 (c) Wound irrigation
 (d) Stress to the wound site
(2) Evaluation measures
 (a) Assess condition of the wound
 (b) Ask whether patient notes any discomfort during procedure
 (c) Inspect condition of dressings at least every shift
(3) Documentation: minimal characteristics in every wound evaluation
 (a) Location
 (b) Size
 (c) Drainage color
 (d) Amount
 (e) Consistency (thick/thin)
 (f) Odor
 (g) NV Status
Continuing Assessment
(1) Monitor vital signs
(2) Monitor distal peripheral pulses
(3) Monitor skin color, sensation and temperature
(4) Monitor motor function
(5) Monitor IV fluids
(6) Provide pain control
(7) Monitor for compartment syndrome
 (a) Pain
 (b) Firmness of muscle compartment
(c) Paresthesia
(8) Evacuate to next echelon of care for further medical treatment as indicated

Wound complications

(1)   Impaired wound healing
         (a)   Accurate observation
         (b)   Ongoing interventions

(2)   Terms associated with wound complications
         (a)   Abscess – Cavity containing pus and surrounded by inflamed tissue, formed as a result of suppuration in a localized infection
         (b)   Adhesion – Band of scar tissue that binds together two anatomical surface normally separated; most commonly found in the abdomen
         (c)   Cellulitis – Infection of the skin characterized by heat, pain, erythema, and edema
         (d)   Dehiscence – Separation of a surgical incision or rupture of a wound closure
         (e)   Evisceration – Protrusion of an internal organ through a wound or surgical incision
         (f)   Extravasation – Passage or escape into the tissues; usually of blood, serum, or lymph
         (g)   Hematoma – Collection of extravasate blood trapped in the tissues or in an organ resulting from incomplete hemostasis after surgery

(3)   Wound bleeding may indicate a slipped suture, dislodged clot, coagulation problem, or trauma placed on blood vessels or tissues

(4)   Inspection of the wound and dressing aids in detecting increase drainage and color changes

(5)   If bleeding occurs internally
         (a)   Dressing may remain dry while the abdominal cavity collects blood
         (b)   Patient will have increase thirst, restlessness, rapid, thready pulse, decreased blood pressure, decreased urinary output, and cool, clammy skin
         (c)   Abdomen will become rigid and distended
         (d)   If not detected, hypovolmic shock can cause circulatory system to collapse, causing death

(6)   Dehiscence – wound layers have separated
         (a)   Patient may say that something has 'given way'
         (b)   May result after periods of sneezing, coughing, or vomiting
         (c)   Evidence of new or increased serosanguineous drainage on the dressing is an important sign to assess
         (d)   Management:
                 (i)   Patient should remain in bed
                 (ii)   Kept NPO
                 (iii)   Told not to cough
                 (iv)   Always reassure patient
                 (v)   Place sterile dressing over area until physician evaluates the site

(7)   Evisceration – abdominal organs protrude through opened incision
         (a)   Patient is to remain in bed

(b)   Wound and contents should be covered up with warm, sterile saline dressings

(c)   Surgeon is notified immediately – this is a medical emergency

(8)   Wound infection, or wound sepsis – results when the surgical wound becomes contaminated

(a)   CDC labels a wound infected when it contains purulent (pus) drainage

(b)   Patient with an infected wound displays a fever, tenderness and pain at the wound, edema, and an elevated WBC

(c)   Purulent drainage has an odor and is brown, yellow or green, depending on the pathogen

TERMINAL LEARNING OBJECTIVE

Give the necessary medical equipment in a holding or ward setting. You are providing casualty care as part of an integrated team in a Minimal Care Ward.

Suctioning Techniques

Suctioning
Used to clear the airway of excessive secretions when the patient is unable to clear the respiratory tract with coughing.

Signs and symptoms of excess secretions
(1)   Assess oral cavity: gurgling noise on inspiration or expiration, obvious oral secretions, drooling, gastric secretions or vomitus in mouth, and productive cough without expectorating secretions from the mouth.

(2)   Assess for lower airway obstruction: coughing, secretions in the airway, labored breathing, restlessness or irritability, unilateral breath sounds, cyanosis, decreased oxygen saturations or level of consciousness, increased fatigue, dizziness, increased pulse rate, increased respiratory rate and/or elevated blood pressure.

Assess lung sounds
Auscultating all lung fields for adventitious sounds such as rhonchi, rales and or wheezing.

Assess the patient's understanding of the procedure
Remove excess secretions by one of the primary suctioning techniques.

Three primary suctioning techniques
(1)   Oropharyngeal suctioning-used when the patient is able to cough effectively but is unable to clear secretions by expectorating or swallowing.

(2)   Nasotracheal suctioning-necessary when the patient with pulmonary secretions is unable to cough and does not have an artificial airway.

(3)   Tracheal suctioning-accomplished through an artificial airway. The artificial airway may be an endotracheal or nasotracheal tube or it may be a tracheostomy tube.

Preparation for all techniques/types of suctioning
(1)   Verify MD/PA order as required for procedure. Some hospitals require a physicians order to suction the trachea

(2)   Explain the procedure to the patient and the reason that it is to be done. Explain how the procedure with help clear the airway and relieve breathing problems and that temporary coughing, sneezing, gagging, or shortness of breath is normal.

(3)   Gather equipment necessary to correctly perform the procedure. Some facilities have commercially prepared suctioning kits. Check what is available in your facility or check procedural manuals for equipment lists.

(4)   Don gloves (nonsterile) and use mask or face shield as per local
        policy
(5)   Fill basin or cup with approximately 100 cc of water
(6)   Connect one end of connecting tubing to suction machine. Check
        that equipment is functioning properly by suctioning a small amount
        of water from basin
(7)   Turn on suction device. Set regulator to appropriate negative
        pressure: wall suction, 80-120 mm Hg; portable suction, 7-15 mm Hg
        for adults

NOTE: Elevated pressure settings increase risk of trauma to mucosa

Oropharyngeal suctioning
(1)   Attach suction catheter to connecting tubing. Remove oxygen mask
        from patient if present. Nasal cannula or prongs may be left in place
        while performing this type of suctioning.
(2)   Assist the patient to assume comfortable position for the procedure.
        Usually this will be a semi-Fowler's position or sitting upright. Proper
        positioning reduces stimulation of the gag reflex, promotes patient
        comfort and aids in secretion drainage.
(3)   Insert catheter into patient's mouth. With suction applied, move the
        catheter around the mouth, including the pharynx and the gum line
        until secretions are cleared. If the catheter does not have a suction
        control to apply intermittent suction, take care not to traumatize oral
        mucosal surfaces with continuous suctioning.

NOTE: Oropharyngeal suctioning is usually performed using a rigid plastic catheter
with one large and several small eyelets that mucous enters when suction is
applied. This type of catheter is called a Yankauer or tonsil suctioning device. Alert
patients can be taught to use this device to control excess secretions in the mouth.

(1)   Encourage the patient to cough. Coughing moves secretions from
        the lower and upper airway into the mouth where they can be easily
        suctioned.
(2)   Repeat suctioning as needed until the mouth is clear of excess
        secretions.
(3)   Replace the oxygen mask if removed earlier.
(4)   Suction water from the basin through the catheter until the catheter is
        cleared of secretions. Clearing secretions from the catheter and the
        tubing before they dry reduces the possibility of transmission of
        microorganisms and insures delivery of accurate suction pressures.
(5)   Place the catheter in a clean, dry area for reuse with the suction
        turned off. If the patient has been taught to use the suction catheter,
        leave the suction on and the catheter within reach of the patient.
(6)   Dispose of water and clean the basin as per policy. Remove your
        gloves and dispose of per local policy.

Nasotracheal suctioning
    (1)   Open suction kit or catheter using aseptic technique. If sterile drape is available, place it across the patient's chest. Do not allow the suction catheter to touch any non sterile surfaces
    (2)   Unwrap or open a sterile basin and place on the bedside table. Be careful not touch the inside of the sterile basin. Fill the basin with approximately 100 cc of sterile Normal Saline (NS).
    (3)   Apply one sterile glove to each hand, or apply non sterile glove to nondominant hand and sterile glove to dominant hand. Attach non sterile suction tubing to sterile catheter, keeping hand holding catheter sterile.
    (4)   Secure catheter to tubing aseptically. Coat distal 2-3 inches of catheter with water-soluble lubricant (K-Y Jelly/Lubricant).
    (5)   Remove oxygen delivery device, if present, with nondominant hand. **Without applying suction** and using the dominant thumb and forefinger, gently, but quickly insert the sterile catheter into either naris during inhalation with a slight downward slant. Do not force the catheter. Try the other naris if insertion meets resistance or is difficult to insert.

NOTE: Never apply suction during insertion. Application of suction pressure while introducing the catheter into the trachea increases risk of damage to the mucosa and increases the risk of hypoxia because the removal of oxygen present in the airway. Remember that the epiglottis is open during inspiration and facilitates insertion of the catheter into the trachea.

    (6)   Insert the catheter approximately 16-20 cm (6 ½-8 inches) in the adult patient. One method of measuring the correct length of catheter to insert is to use the distance from the patient's nose to the base of the earlobe as a guide.
    (7)   Apply intermittent suction by placing and releasing nondominant thumb over the vent of catheter. Slowly withdraw the catheter while rotating it back and forth with suction on for as long as 10-15 seconds.
    (8)   Assess the need to repeat suctioning procedure. Allow adequate time between suction passes for ventilation and oxygenation. Ask the patient to deep breathe and cough. Keep oxygen readily available in case the patient exhibits signs of hypoxemia. Administer oxygen to the patient between suctioning attempts
    (9)   When the pharynx and trachea are cleared of secretions, perform oral suctioning to clear the mouth of secretions. Do not suction the nose or trachea after suctioning the mouth.
    (10)   Rinse the catheter and connecting tubing by suctioning NS from the basin until the tubing is clear. Dispose of equipment as per facility policy. Turn off suction device

Endotracheal or tracheostomy tube suctioning
    (1)   Performed through an artificial airway (endotracheal/nasotracheal or tracheostomy). Artificial airways are indicated for patients with deceased level of consciousness, airway obstruction, mechanical

ventilation and for removal of tracheal bronchial secretions. Artificial airways allow easy access to the patient's trachea for deep tracheal suctioning.

(2)   Prepare suction equipment, suction catheter using sterile technique and don sterile gloves as previously described for nasotracheal suctioning

(3)   Hyper oxygenate the patient before suctioning, using manual resuscitation Ambu-bag connected to an oxygen source.

(4)   Open swivel adapter or if necessary remove the oxygen delivery device (ventilator tubing) with your nondominant hand.

(5)   **Without applying suction**, gently, but quickly insert the sterile catheter using the dominant thumb and forefinger into the artificial airway until resistance is met, or the patient coughs and them pull back the catheter approximately ½ inch.

(6)   Apply intermittent suction by placing and releasing nondominant thumb over the vent of the catheter while rotating it back and forth between the dominant thumb and forefinger. Encourage the patient to cough, if possible. Observe continuously for respiratory distress.

NOTE: If the patient develops respiratory distress during the suctioning procedure, immediately withdraw the catheter and administer additional oxygen and breaths as needed.

(7)   Close the swivel adapter, or replace the oxygen delivery device (ventilator tubing).

(8)   Rinse catheter and tubing with NS

(9)   Assess for secretion clearance. Repeat suctioning procedure 1-2 times more to clear secretions if necessary. Allow adequate time between suction passes (at least one full minute) for ventilation and oxygenation.

(10)   Perform oropharyngeal suctioning as needed. Catheter is now contaminated. **Do not** reinsert into the artificial airway.

(11)   Dispose of suctioning equipment per policy. Turn off suction device

(14)   Reposition the patient as indicated by condition

Record-
The amount, consistency, color and any odor of secretions and the patient's response to the procedure. Document the patient's pre- and post suctioning respiratory status.

Continue to monitor patient's vital signs
Include pulse oximetry if available.

Perform Endotracheal Tube and Tracheostomy Care

Artificial airways
Place the patient at high risk for infection and make the patient more susceptible to airway injury.

Endotracheal (ET) tubes

Used as short-term artificial airways and are used to administer mechanical ventilation, relieve upper airway obstruction, and protect the patient from aspiration or clear excessive secretions. ET tubes may be placed either nasally or orally. They are generally removed within 14 days.

Patients who require artificial airway assistance for longer than 14 days usually require a tracheostomy. This procedure involves a surgical incision to be made into the trachea and a short, artificial airway (trach tube) is inserted. This procedure is normally accomplished in the operating room under sterile conditions.

Endotracheal (ET) tube care

(1)   Verify MD/PA order as required by facility
(2)   Explain the procedure to the patient and reason it is being done in terms the patient understands
(3)   Gather equipment necessary to perform the procedure
(4)   Initiate and perform endotracheal suctioning prior to the procedure. This allows for the removal of secretion and diminishes the patient's need to cough during the procedure.
(5)   Connect oral suction catheter (Yankauer) suction to suction device
(6)   Prepare tape. Cut piece of tape long enough to go completely around the patient's head from nares to nares (nasal ET tube) or from edge of mouth to edge of mouth (for oral ET tube) plus approximately 6 inches. Lay adhesive side up on table and cut and lay approximately 6 inches of tape, adhesive side down, in the center of the long strip. This will prevent the longer piece of tape from sticking to the patient's skin and hair on the back of the head/neck.
(7)   Carefully remove tape from the ET tube and the patient's face. An assistant may be required to help hold the ET tube in place so that the tube does not move. This is especially important in an uncooperative patient.
(8)   Remove excess adhesive from the face with adhesive remover if necessary.
(9)   Remove bite block or oral airway if present
(10)   Clean mouth, gums and teeth with NS or mouthwash solution and a 4 X 4 gauze, sponge tipped applicator or saline swabs. Brush teeth if necessary and suction oral cavity with Yankauer suction.
(11)   Clean face and neck with soap and water. Shave the make client as necessary.
(12)   Apply tincture of benzoin to the upper lip (oral ET tube) or across nose (nasal ET tube) and cheeks to ears. Allow to dry completely.
(13)   Slip tape under the patient's head and neck, adhesive side down. Do not twist tape or catch hair. Do not allow tape to stick to itself. Center tape so that the double-faced tape extends around the back of the neck from ear to ear.
(14)   On one side of the face, secure tape from ear to nares (nasal ET tube) or edge of mouth (oral ET tube). Tear remaining tape in half, length wise, forming two pieces that are ½ to ¾ inch wide. Secure

bottom half of tape across upper lip (oral ET tube) or across tope of nose (nasal ET tube). Wrap top half around the ET tube.
(15)   Gently pull other side of tape firmly to pick up slack and secure to remaining side of face.
(16)   Clean oral airway in warm soapy water and rinse well. Hydrogen peroxide can aid in the removal of crusty secretions.
(14)   Reinsert oral airway being careful not to push the tongue into the oropharnyx

Tacheostomy Care
(1)   Suction trach. Suctioning prior to the procedure removes secretions so that they do not occlude the outer cannula while the inner cannula is removed. Reduces the need for the patient to cough during the procedure.
(2)   Open sterile trach care kit (commercially available). Open three 4 X 4 sterile gauze packages using aseptic technique and pour NS on one package and hydrogen peroxide on another. Leave the third package dry.
(3)   Open two packages of cotton tipped swabs and pour NS on one package and hydrogen peroxide on the other.
(4)   Open sterile trach package. Unwrap sterile basin and pour about 1 inch of hydrogen peroxide into it. Open small sterile brush package and place aseptically into the basin.
(5)   Measure and cut twill trach tape long enough to around the patient's neck two times (approximately 24-30 inches. Cut ends on a diagonal. Lay aside in a dry area.
(6)   Don sterile gloves. Keep dominant hand sterile throughout the procedure.
(7)   Remove oxygen source/ventilator tubing.
(8)   Remove inner cannula of trach with a slight twisting motion with the nondominant hand and drop the cannula into the hydrogen peroxide basin
(9)   Place oxygen source over or near the outer cannula. Oxygen delivery tubing cannot be attached to all outer cannulas when the inner cannula is removed.
(10)   Quickly clean the inner cannula with the brush to remove secretions inside and outside the cannula. Rinse with NS, using the nondominant hand to pour.
(11)   Replace the inner cannula and secure the locking mechanism with a slight twisting motion. Reapply the oxygen/ventilator source.
(12)   Using hydrogen peroxide prepared cotton-tipped swabs and 4 X 4 gauze, clean the outer cannula surfaces and stoma under the faceplate of the trach tube, extending 2-4 inches in all directions from the stoma. Clean in a circular motion from stoma site outward. Always remember to use the dominant hand to handle sterile supplies
(13)   Using NS prepared cotton-tipped swabs and 4 X 4 gauze, rinse hydrogen peroxide from the trach tube and skin.
(14)   Using dry 4 X 4 gauze, pat dry the outer cannula and skin surfaces.

(15)   Replace trach tie. If assistant available, have them hold the trach in place while old tie is cut and removed and new tie is applied. If no assistant is available, apply new tie before removing the old one.
(16)   To replace the trach tie, insert one end of the tie through faceplate eyelet and pull ends even
(17)   Slide both ends of behind the head and around the neck to the other eyelet and insert one tie through the second eyelet.
(18)   Pull snug
(19)   Tie ends securely in a double square knot, allowing space for only one finger in tie
(20)   Insert fresh trach dressing under clean ties and faceplate.
(21)   Assist patient to position of comfort and assess respiratory status.

Record respiratory assessments before and after care.

Record ET tube care-
Include frequency and extent of care, patient response to care and any abnormal findings to include skin breakdown/irritation.

Record tracheostomy care-.
Note size of trach tube, frequency and extent of care, patient tolerance of care and any abnormal findings to include signs of an infected stoma (increased redness, purulent drainage), skin breakdown/irritation.

Continue to monitor patient's vital signs-
Include pulse oximetry, if available.

Administer a nebulization treatment

Nebulization
Process of adding moisture or medications to inspired air by mixing particles of varying size using compressed air or oxygen.

Nebulizer-
Uses the aerosol principle to suspend a maximum number of water drops or particles of the desired size in inspired air.

Nebulization-
Often used for the administration of bronchodilator in the treatment of asthma

Administer a nebulization treatment
(1)   Verify MD/PA order for treatment
(2)   Verify patient's allergies to medications
(3)   Prepare medication. Usually administer a bronchodilator such as albuterol, 0.2-0.3 ml in 3cc normal saline (NS). This medication is often available in unit dose packages. Check with facility for what is available.
(4)   Assemble nebulizer as directed. Nebulizers are now pre-packaged, disposable systems for individual patient use.

(5)   Place medication and NS into receptacle and screw lid onto medication receptacle. Attach the mouthpiece to the receptacle and attach the reservoir tubing to the other end.

(6)   Connect the nebulizer to the compressed air or oxygen source. Oxygen is usually used to administer a nebulization treatment to a patient having an acute asthmatic attack.

(7)   Turn on the compressed air/oxygen until you observe a fine mist coming from the mouthpiece of the nebulizer. This usually requires at least 10-12 LPM of the compressed air/oxygen.

(8)   Have the patient place the mouthpiece in their mouth and close their lips around the mouthpiece.

(9)   Patient should inhale the medication as deeply as possible and exhale through the nebulizer. The patient does not need to remove the nebulizer from their mouth to exhale. Make sure the patient does not hyperventilate nor hold his breath.

(10)   The treatment should last 5-10 minutes.

(11)   Upon completion of the treatment, turn off the compressed air/oxygen.

(12)   Assess the respiratory status of the patient by auscultating the lungs

(13)   Monitor vital signs to include pulse oximetry if available

(14)   Document the treatment to include time, medication, deliver system and patient's response to treatment.

TERMINAL LEARNING OBJECTIVE

Give the necessary medical equipment in a holding or ward setting.   You are providing casualty care as part of an integrated team in a Minimal Care Ward, perform basic nursing care IAW *Advanced Cardiac Life Support*, *Emergency Medicine*, *Nursing Interventions and Clinical Skills*.

Basic Cardiac Monitoring
   Electrocardiogram (ECG)

(1)	Graphic record of heart's electrical activity
(2)	Body acts a conductor of electricity and the heart is the largest generator of electrical energy
(3)	Electrodes placed on the skin can detect total electrical activity within the heart
(4)	Electrical impulses on the skin surface have very low voltage. The ECG machine amplifies these impulses and records them on the ECG graph paper or on a monitor screen called an oscilloscope.
(5)	Positive impulses appear as "upward" deflections on the graph paper or monitor screen
(6)	Negative impulses appear as "downward" deflection on the graph paper or monitor screen
(7)	Absence of any electrical impulse produces an isoelectric or "flat" line
(8)	"Artifacts" are deflections the ECG produced by factors other than the electrical activity of the heart. Common causes are:
	(a) Muscle tremors
	(b) Shivering
	(c) Patient movement
	(d) Loose electrodes
	(e) 60 cycle interference
	(f) Machine malfunction
(9)	Eliminate all artifacts before attempting to record an ECG
	(a) Replace loose electrodes
	(b) Cover patient with a blanket to prevent shivering
	(c) Wipe oily skin or diaphoretic skin with alcohol and then attach leads to increase adherence to the skin

   ECG Leads

(1)	Monitors heart's electrical activity by monitoring voltage change through electrodes placed at various places on the body surface
(2)	Each pair of electrodes is called a "lead"
(3)	Basic cardiac monitoring uses only 3 leads
(4)	Three types of ECG leads are:
	(a) Bipolar
	(b) Augmented
	(c) Precordial
(5)	Bipolar leads are the most frequently used and have one positive electrode and one negative electrode

(6)   Leads I, II and III commonly called limb leads are bipolar and are the most frequently used leads in basic cardiac monitoring

NOTE: In the definitive care facility, 12 leads are normally used to detect a variety of conduction abnormalities, to include the presence and location of a myocardial infarction. This technique requires the use of augmented limb leads and precordial leads and allows the examination of the heart in two planes.

(7)   Bipolar leads provide only three views of the heart's electrical activity, which is adequate for detecting life-threatening dysrhythmias

Routine ECG Monitoring

(1)   Routine ECG monitoring generally uses only one lead
(2)   Most commonly monitored leads are either Lead II or the modified chest lead 1 (MCL1),
(3)   Lead II is used more frequently because most of the heart's electrical current flows toward its positive axis. This lead gives the best view of the ECG waves and best shows the heart's conduction system's activity.

NOTE: MCL is a special monitoring lead that some systems use selectively to help determine the origin of abnormal complexes such as premature beats.

Lead Placement

(1)   Electrodes are place on the chest wall
(2)   Positive lead is placed at the apex of the heart-usually a few inches below the left nipple. Often the leads are marked for placement, RA (right arm), LA (left arm), etc.
(3)   The negative electrode is place below the right clavicle
(4)   The third electrode, the ground, is place somewhere on the left upper chest wall, usually below the left clavicle

Advantages of single lead monitoring:

(1)   Simple system
(2)   Provides rate of the heartbeat
(3)   Provides regularity of the heartbeat
(4)   Provides conduction time of the impulse through the heart
(5)   Detects life threatening dysrhythmias

Disadvantages of single lead monitoring

(1)   Does not provide the presence or location of an infarct
(2)   Does not provide right-to-left differences in conduction or impulse formation

(3)   Does not provide information on the quality or presence of pumping
        action

Perform a 12 Lead ECG

Check equipment

(1)   Ensure machine is turned on and allow ample time to warm up
(2)   Inspect machine for any malfunctions
(3)   Check machine's paper supply
(4)   Ensure all equipment is on hand
        (a)   Diskette
        (b)   Clean electrodes

Gather information for Electrocardiogram Report

(1)   Patient age
(2)   Patient sex
(3)   Race
(4)   Weight
(5)   Height
(6)   Signature of requesting MD/PA
(7)   Date and time of recording
(8)   Patient diagnosis or reason for recording
(9)   Current medications
(10)   Previous ECGs
(11)   Priority of processing
(12)   Patient identification
        (a)   Patient name and rank
        (b)   Social security number
        (c)   Company assignment if active duty
        (d)   Home phone number if retired

Procedure for recording a standard 12-lead ECG

(1)   Explain procedure to the patient
(2)   Select electrode sites
        (a)   Arms - anterior forearm and biceps
        (b)   Legs - medial aspect of lower leg
        (c)   Chest positions
                (i)   V1 - fourth intercostal space, right sternal
                (ii)   V2 - fourth intercostal space, left sternal
                (iii)   V3 - midway between V2 and V4
                (iv)   V4 - fifth intercostal space, midclavicular line
                (v)   V5 - same level as V4, anterior axillary line
                (vi)   V6 - same level as V4 and V5, midaxillary line
        (d)   Special cases of placement
                (i)   Amputees - place lead proximal to stump
                (ii)   Hairy skin surface - if hair is excessive, rub with
                        alcohol

        (iii)   Female - place lead under breast
        (iv)   Exceptionally oily skin - rub with alcohol
        (v)   Hard or scaly skin - rub with alcohol
        (vi)   Parkinson's disease
                *   Place electrode high on limb
                *   Elevating extremities in resting position may help control shaking
        (vii)   Skin rashes
                *   Find area without a rash
                *   If possible, rub with alcohol
        (viii)   Metal particles embedded in skin - move electrode site

(3)   Wipe selected area with alcohol before applying electrode
(4)   Application of electrodes
        (a)   Ensure electrodes are not falling off patient
        (b)   Ensure patient cable is not twisted and not interfering with other leads
        (c)   Select flat, fleshy site on arms and legs, avoid bone
(5)   Press record ECG button
        (a)   Remind patient to relax
        (b)   Check leads for contact
(6)   Recognize a good ECG
        (a)   Sharp distinct baseline
        (b)   Free from artifact
        (c)   Centered on graph
(7)   Disconnect ECG
        (a)   Disconnect patient
        (b)   Clean electrode surfaces as you remove them from the patient

Identify general problems

(1)   Muscle tremor
        (a)   Causes
                (i)   Patient uncomfortable or cold
                (ii)   60-cycle interference
        (b)   Correction
                (i)   Ensure patient comfort. Provide a cover if room is cold.
                (ii)   Ensure patient is not holding anything in their hand
                (iii)   Ensure feet are not touching the wall or foot board
(2)   60-cycle interference
        (a)   Causes
                (i)   Ungrounded electrocardiograph
                (ii)   Ungrounded electrical outlet
                (iii)   Ungrounded equipment that is connected to same electrical outlet
        (b)   Correction

              (i)   Change electrical outlets
              (ii)   Change electrocardiograph, if possible
              (iii)   Notify MD/PA and medical maintenance

(3)   Wandering baseline
     (a)   Causes
              (i)   Poor electrode contact
              (ii)   Cable pulling on electrodes
              (iii)   Cable moving with respirations
     (b)   Correction
              (i)   Check electrodes to ensure good contact
              (ii)   Adjust patient cable and move
                      electrocardiograph closer to patient
              (iii)   Move cable off abdomen and guide under
                      patient's arm to stabilize from moving

Right Side and Posterior ECG's

Right side and Posterior ECG's are recorded to aid the MD/PA in diagnosing the location of a myocardial infarction

(1)   Explain the procedure to the patient
(2)   Select electrode sites
     (a)   Chest positions: V3R - 6R, are placed on the right side of the chest in the same locations as the Left side leads V3-6 would be placed. V2R is therefore the same as V1
              (i)   V1R - fourth intercostal space, left sternal border
              (ii)   V2R - fourth intercostal space, Right sternal border
              (iii)   V3R - midway between V2R and V4R
              (iv)   V4R - fifth intercostal space, midclavicular line
              (v)   V5R - same level as V4R, anterior axillary line
              (vi)   V6R - same level as V4R and V5R, midaxillary line
     (b)   All other preparation and clean up steps of the procedure remain the same as for standard 12-lead ECG

Posterior ECG's

(1)   Explain the procedure to the patient
(2)   Select electrode sites
     (a)   Leads for a posterior ECG are placed in a horizontal line across the back
     (b)   Back Positions: May be done with standard left-side ECG - V7, 8, 9 or with Right-sided ECG - V7R, 8R, 9R
              (i)   V7 - Posterior axillary line
              (ii)   V8 - Posterior Scapular line
              (iii)   V9 - Left border of the spine
              (iv)   V7R - Right posterior axillary line
              (v)   V8R - Right posterior scapular line
              (vi)   V9R - Right border of the spine

(c)   All other preparation and clean up steps of the procedure
        remain the same as for standard 12-lead ECG

Measure Pulse Oxygen Saturation
Pulse oximetry defined

(1)   Noninvasive measurement of arterial oxygen saturation
(2)   Assess level of oxygen in the blood available to the body tissues
(3)   Reflects percent of hemoglobin that is bound with oxygen in the
        arteries
(4)   Expressed as a percentage
        (a)   For example, 96% indicates 96% of the hemoglobin
                molecules are carrying oxygen molecules
        (b)   The more hemoglobin is saturated, the higher the
                percentage
        (c)   Normally over 90%
        (d)   An arterial blood gas (ABG) is an invasive procedure that
                may also be used to measure arterial oxygen saturation
(5)   Pulse oximetry is accurate to +/- 2% for all readings over 70%
(6)   Pulse oximetry is simple, painless, and has fewer risks than
        obtaining an ABG

Pulse oximeter - how it works

(1)   Probe with a light-emitting diode (LED) connected by cable to an
        oximeter
(2)   Light waves emitted by LED are absorbed and reflected back by
        oxygenated and deoxygenated hemoglobin molecules
(3)   Reflected light is processed by the oximeter, which calculated the
        arterial oxygen saturation
(4)   The oximeter sensor probe is applied to:
        (a)   Finger
        (b)   Toe
        (c)   Earlobe
        (d)   Bridge of the nose

Considerations

(1)   Patients at risk for unstable oxygen status
        (a)   Acute respiratory disease
        (b)   Chronic respiratory disease
        (c)   Ventilator dependence
        (d)   Chest pain
        (e)   Activity intolerance
        (f)   Recovery from general anesthesia
        (g)   Recovery from conscious sedation
        (h)   Traumatic injury to chest wall
        (i)   Changes in supplemental oxygen therapy
(2)   Medications or treatments that may influence oxygen saturation
        (a)   Oxygen therapy

           (b)   Respiratory therapy

(3)   Factors that influence oxygen saturation - abnormalities in type of amount of hemoglobin affect the ability of oxygen to be carried to the tissues

(4)   Factors likely to interfere with accuracy of pulse oximeter
        (a)   Skin pigmentation - darker pigments can result in false-high readings
        (b)   Jaundice
        (c)   Intravascular dyes

(5)   Assess pertinent laboratory values, including hemoglobin and ABGs if available
        (a)   Anemia affects ability of oxygen to attach to hemoglobin molecule
        (b)   ABGs measure arterial oxygen saturation, which serves as a standard and provides a basis for comparison

(6)   Determine client-specific sit appropriate to place pulse oximeter probe by measuring capillary refill
        (a)   Site must have adequate circulation
        (b)   Moisture, dark nail polish, and acrylic nails impede sensor detection of emitted light and produce falsely elevated arterial oxygen saturation levels

(7)   Determine previous baseline from patient's records

Application of pulse oximeter

(1)   Select site and determine capillary refill
(2)   Attach sensor probe to selected site
(3)   Turn on oximeter
        (a)   Observe pulse waveform/intensity display
        (b)   Compare oximeter pulse rate with client's radial pulse
(4)   Once oximeter reaches constant value, read arterial oxygen saturation on display
(5)   Continually monitor arterial oxygen saturation levels
(6)   Notify MD/PA of drastic changes

TERMINAL LEARNING OBJECTIVE

Give the necessary medical equipment in a holding or ward setting. You are providing casualty care as part of an integrated team in a Minimal Care Ward. Performed basic nursing care for casualty without causing further injury or illness.

Chest Tube Systems

Pleur-Evac chest drainage system
(1)   One-piece molded plastic unit that duplicates the three-bottle system
(2)   Cost effective
(3)   There must be bubbles flowing in the suction control portion of the unit to provide suction to the patient

Pleur-Evac Set Up
(1)   Fill water seal chamber
(2)   Fill suction control chamber
(3)   Attach tube to suction source
(4)   Tape all the connections
(5)   Provide sterile tube for connection to patient

Procedure for Proper Usage of the Heimlich Valve
(1)   Heimlich valve is a plastic, portable one-way valve used for chest drainage, draining into a vented bag
(2)   Equipment
    (a)   Heimlich valve
    (b)   Kelly clamps - 2 (rubber-tipped)
    (c)   Vented drainage bag or ostomy bag
    (d)   Ostomy tape or rubber band
    (e)   Suction setup (if applicable)
    (f)   Clean scissors
(3)   Procedure Steps
    (a)   Gather equipment and bring to patient area
    (b)   Wash hands
    (c)   Don gloves. Nonsterile gloves are acceptable as long as sterile technique is maintained while the connection is being made.
(4)   Heimlich Valve To Chest Tube
    (a)   Place rubber-tipped Kelly clamps in opposite directions on the proximal end of the chest tube as near to the patient as possible
    (b)   Connect the chest tube to the blue end of the Heimlich valve using sterile technique

CAUTION: Only the blue end of the Heimlich valve can be connected to the chest tube. If the clear end is connected, the one-way valve will be in the wrong position and no drainage will take place.

    (c)   Tape the connection site at both ends of the valve using 2 inch cloth tape.

CAUTION: When two chest tubes are present, two Heimlich valves must be used to ensure proper functioning of chest tubes.

(d)   Monitor and record character of drainage and patency of valve in nursing progress notes.

CAUTION: Measure all drainage in a calibrated cylinder for accurate readings.

(e)   Record drainage output on I & O graphic every 8 hours. If conditions permit.

Care of patients with chest tubes

Assess patient for respiratory distress and chest pain, breath sounds over affected lung area, and stable vital signs

Observe for increase respiratory distress

Observe the following:
(1)   Chest tube dressing, ensure tubing is patent
(2)   Tubing kinks, dependent loops or clots
(3)   Chest drainage system, which should be upright and below level of tube insertion

Provide two shodded hemostats for each chest tube, attached to top of patient's bed with adhesive tape. Chest tubes are only clamped under specific circumstances:
(1)   To assess air leak
(2)   To quickly empty or change collection bottle or chamber; performed by soldier medic who has received training in procedure
(3)   To change disposable systems; have new system ready to be connected before clamping tube so that transfer can be rapid and drainage system reestablished
(4)   To change a broken water-seal bottle in the event that no sterile solution container is available
(5)   To assess if patient is ready to have chest tube removed (which is done by physician's order); the solider medic must monitor patient for recreation of pneumothorax

Position the patient to permit optimal drainage
(1)   Semi-Flower's position to evacuate air (pneumothorax)
(2)   High Flower's position to drain fluid (hemothorax)

Maintain tube connection between chest and drainage tubes intact and taped
(1)   Water-seal vent must be without occlusion
(2)   Suction-control chamber vent must be without occlusion when suction is used

Coil excess tubing on mattress next to patient. Secure with rubber band and safety pin or system's clamp

Adjust tubing to hang in straight line from top of mattress to drainage chamber. If chest tube is draining fluid, indicate time (e.g., 0900) that drainage was begun on drainage bottle's adhesive tape or on write-on surface of disposable commercial system
(1)   Strip or milk chest tube only per MD/PA orders only
(2)   Follow local policy for this procedure

Problems solving with chest tubes

Problem: Air leak
(1)   Problem: Continuous bubbling is seen in water-seal bottle/chamber, indicating that leak is between patient and water seal
         (a)   Locate leak
         (b)   Tighten loose connection between patient and water seal
         (c)   Loose connections cause air to enter system.
         (d)   Leaks are corrected when constant bubbling stops
(2)   Problem: Bubbling continues, indicating that air leak has not been corrected
         (a)   Cross-clamp chest tube close to patient's chest, if bubbling stops, air leak is inside the patient's thorax or at chest tube insertion site
         (b)   Unclamp tube and notify physician immediately!
         (c)   Reinforce chest dressing

Warning: Leaving chest tube clamped caused a tension pneumothorax and mediastinal shift

(3)   Problem: Bubbling continues, indicating that leak is not in the patient's chest or at the insertion site
         (a)   Gradually move clamps down drainage tubing away from patient and toward suction-control chamber, moving one clamp at a time
         (b)   When bubbling stops, leak is in section of tubing or connection distal to the clamp
         (c)   Replace tubing or secure connection and release clamp
(4)   Problem: Bubbling continues, indicating that leak is not in tubing
         (a)   Leak is in drainage system
         (b)   Change drainage system

Problem: Tension pneumothorax is present
(1)   Problems: Severe respiratory distress or chest pain
         (a)   Determine that chest tubes are not clamped, kinked, or occluded. Locate leak
         (b)   Obstructed chest tubes trap air in intrapleural space when air leak originates within patient
(2)   Problem: Absence of breath sounds on affected side
         (a)   Notify physician immediately

(3)   Problems: Hyperresonance on affected side, mediastinal shift to unaffected side, tracheal shift to unaffected side, hyptenstion or tachycardia
      (a)   Immediately prepare for another chest tube insertion
      (b)   Obtain a flutter (Heimlich) valve or large-guage needle for short-term emergency release or air in intrapleural space
      (c)   Have emergency equipment (oxygen and code cart) near patient

(4)   Problem: Dependent loops of drainage tubing have trapped fluid
      (a)   Drain tubing contents into drainage bottle
      (b)   Coil excess tubing on mattress and secure in place

(5)   Problem: Water seal is disconnected
      (a)   Connect water seal
      (b)   Tape connection

(6)   Problem: Water-seal bottle is broken
      (a)   Insert distal end of water-seal tube into sterile solution so that tip is 2 cm below surface
      (b)   Set up new water-seal bottle
      (c)   If no sterile solution is available, double clamp chest tube while preparing new bottle

(7)   Problem: Water-seal tube is no longer submerged in sterile fluid
      (a)   Add sterile solution to water-seal bottle until distal tip is 2 cm under surface
      (b)   Or set water-seal bottle upright so that tip is submerged

Appendix A
Wound Care
Competency Skill Sheets

Irrigation

Soldiers Name: _____ SSN: _____ CO: _____ TM: _____
Start: _____ Stop: _____ Initial Evaluator: _____
Start: _____ Stop: _____ Retest Evaluator: _____
Start: _____ Stop: _____ Final Evaluator: _____

		1st	2nd	3rd
a.	Identifies patient and explains procedure to patient.	P / F	P / F	P / F
b.	Performs patient care handwash.	P / F	P / F	P / F
c.	Assembles equipment needed.	P / F	P / F	P / F
d.	Positions and drapes patient as necessary.	P / F	P / F	P / F
e.	Positions waterproof pad under wound.	P / F	P / F	P / F
f.	Establishes a sterile field.	P / F	P / F	P / F
g.	Dons gown and goggles as appropriate.	P / F	P / F	P / F
h.	Dons clean gloves, removes dressing and discards.	P / F	P / F	P / F
i.	Assesses wound prior to irrigation, noting size, color, warmth, and amount of discharge or blood from wound.	P / F	P / F	P / F
j.	Removes gloves and performs a patient care handwash.	P / F	P / F	P / F
k.	Dons sterile gloves.	P / F	P / F	P / F
l.	Cleans area around wound.	P / F	P / F	P / F
m.	Fills irrigating syringe with solution; attach a soft catheter if needed for a deep wound with a small opening.	P / F	P / F	P / F
n.	Instills solution gently into wound, holding syringe 1" above wound. If using a catheter, gently insert into the wound opening until slight resistance is met, pull back and gently instills solution.	P / F	P / F	P / F
o.	Allows solution to flow from clean area of wound to dirty area.	P / F	P / F	P / F
p.	Refills solution and continue irrigation until solution return is clear.	P / F	P / F	P / F
q.	Blots wound edges with sterile gauze.	P / F	P / F	P / F
r.	Redresses wound.	P / F	P / F	P / F
s.	Removes gloves and all equipment, discarding in appropriate biohazard receptacles as required.	P / F	P / F	P / F
t.	Performs patient care handwash.	P / F	P / F	P / F
u.	Documents procedure.	P / F	P / F	P / F
v.	Verbalizes that he/she would report an increase in pain, fresh bleeding, retention of irrigant solution or sings of shock to MD/PA.	P / F	P / F	P / F

Instructor Comments:

Sterile Field

Soldiers Name: _____ SSN: _____ CO: _____ TM: _____
Start: _____ Stop: _____ Initial Evaluator: _____
Start: _____ Stop: _____ Retest Evaluator: _____
Start: _____ Stop: _____ Final Evaluator: _____

		1st	2nd	3rd
a.	Selects clean work surface above waist level.	P / F	P / F	P / F
b.	Assembles necessary equipment.	P / F	P / F	P / F
c.	Checks dates, labels and condition of packaging for sterility of equipment.	P / F	P / F	P / F
d.	Performs patient care handwash.	P / F	P / F	P / F
e.	Places pack directly on work surface and opens as described to ensure sterility of the sterile drape.	P / F	P / F	P / F
f.	Gently lifts drape up from its outer cover and lets it unfold by itself without touching any object; discards outer cover with the other hand.	P / F	P / F	P / F
g.	Grasps adjacent corner of drape and holds it straight up and away from body; now drape is properly places while using two hands. Drape must be held away unsterile surface.	P / F	P / F	P / F
h.	Holding drape, first positions the bottom half over the intended work surface.	P / F	P / F	P / F
i.	Allows top half of drape to be placed over work surface last.	P / F	P / F	P / F
j.	Performs procedure using sterile technique.	P / F	P / F	P / F

Instructor Comments:

Appendix B
Cardiac Monitoring
Competency Skill Sheets

Pulse Ox

Soldiers Name: _____ SSN: _____ CO: _____ TM: _____
Start: _____ Stop: _____ Initial Evaluator: _____
Start: _____ Stop: _____ Retest Evaluator: _____
Start: _____ Stop: _____ Final Evaluator: _____

		1st	2nd	3rd
a.	Selected site. If finger is selected, removed fingernail polish or acrylic nail.	P / F	P / F	P / F
b.	Determined capillary refill at site. If less than 3 seconds, selected alternative site.	P / F	P / F	P / F
c.	Position patient comfortably. (1) Supported lower arm if finger is chosen as monitoring site. (2) Instructed client to keep sensor probe site still.	P / F	P / F	P / F
d.	Attached sensor probe to selected site. Ensured photo detectors of light sensors are aligned opposite each other.	P / F	P / F	P / F
e.	Turned on oximeter by activating power. (1) Observed pulse waveform/intensity display and audible beep. (2) Compared oximeter pulse rate with patient's radial pulse.	P / F	P / F	P / F
f.	Left sensor probe in place until oximeter reaches constant value and pulse display reaches full strength.	P / F	P / F	P / F
g.	Read SpO2 on digital display.	P / F	P / F	P / F
h.	Checked SpO2 alarm limits, if continues SpO2 monitoring is planned . (1) Determined limits for SpO2 and pulse rate as indicated by patient's condition. (2) Verified alarms are on. (3) Relocated sensor probe every 4 hours (if indicated).	P / F	P / F	P / F
i.	Removed probe and turned off oximeter power.	P / F	P / F	P / F

Instructor Comments:

12 Lead EKG

Soldiers Name: _____ SSN: _____ CO: _____ TM: _____
Start: _____ Stop: _____ Initial Evaluator: _____
Start: _____ Stop: _____ Retest Evaluator: _____
Start: _____ Stop: _____ Final Evaluator: _____

		1st	2nd	3rd
a.	Checked equipment.	P / F	P / F	P / F
	(1) Ensured machine is turned on and allowed ample time to warm up.			
	(2) Inspected machine for any malfunctions.			
	(3) Checked machine's paper supply.			
	(4) Ensured all equipment is on hand.			
b.	Gathered patient information.	P / F	P / F	P / F
c.	Explained procedure to the patient.	P / F	P / F	P / F
d.	Selected electrode site (arms, legs, and chest positions).	P / F	P / F	P / F
e.	Considered special cases of placement.	P / F	P / F	P / F
f.	Wiped selected area with alcohol before applying electrode.	P / F	P / F	P / F
g.	Applied electrodes.	P / F	P / F	P / F
	(1) Ensured electrodes are not falling off patient.			
	(2) Ensured patient cable is not twisted and not interfering with other leads.			
h.	Pressed record EKG button.	P / F	P / F	P / F
	(1) Reminded patient to relax.			
	(2) Checked leads for contact.			
i.	Recognized a good EKG.	P / F	P / F	P / F
j.	Disconnected EKG.	P / F	P / F	P / F
	(1) Disconnected patient.			
	(2) Cleaned electrode surfaces as removed from patient.			

Instructor Comments:

Appendix C
Respiratory Care
Competency Skill Sheets

Nebulization

Soldiers Name: _____ SSN: _____ CO: _____ TM: _____
Start: _____ Stop: _____ Initial Evaluator: _____
Start: _____ Stop: _____ Retest Evaluator: _____
Start: _____ Stop: _____ Final Evaluator: _____

		1st	2nd	3rd
a.	Verified MD/PA order for treatment.	P / F	P / F	P / F
b.	Verified patient's allergies to medication.	P / F	P / F	P / F
c.	Prepared medication.	P / F	P / F	P / F
d.	Assembled nebulizer as directed.	P / F	P / F	P / F
e.	Placed medication and NS into receptacle. Screwed lid onto medication receptacle.	P / F	P / F	P / F
f.	Attached mouthpiece to receptacle. Attached reservoir tubing to other end.	P / F	P / F	P / F
g.	Connected nebulizer to compressed air or oxygen source.	P / F	P / F	P / F
h.	Turned on compressed air/oxygen until a fine mist is observed from mouthpiece of nebulizer (usually requires 10-12 LPM of compressed air/oxygen).	P / F	P / F	P / F
i.	Had patient place mouthpiece in mouth and close lips around mouthpiece.	P / F	P / F	P / F
j.	Instructed patient to inhale medication as deeply as possible and exhale through nebulizer. (1) Made sure patient did not hyperventilate or hold breath.	P / F	P / F	P / F
k.	Allowed treatment 5-10 minutes.	P / F	P / F	P / F
l.	Upon completion of treatment, turned off compressed air/oxygen.	P / F	P / F	P / F
m.	Assessed respiratory status by auscultating the lungs.	P / F	P / F	P / F
n.	Monitored vital signs, including pulse oximetry (if available).	P / F	P / F	P / F
o.	Documented treatment.	P / F	P / F	P / F

Instructor Comments:

Inhaler

Soldiers Name: _____ SSN: _____ CO: _____ TM: _____
Start: _____ Stop: _____ Initial Evaluator: _____
Start: _____ Stop: _____ Retest Evaluator: _____
Start: _____ Stop: _____ Final Evaluator: _____

		1st	2nd	3rd
a.	Verified MD/PA orders.	P / F	P / F	P / F
b.	Assessed patient's ability to hold, manipulate, and depress inhaler.	P / F	P / F	P / F
c.	Assessed patient's knowledge and understanding of purpose and action of prescribed inhaler.	P / F	P / F	P / F
d.	Assessed drug schedule and number of inhalations prescribed for each dose.	P / F	P / F	P / F
e.	Positioned patient comfortably.	P / F	P / F	P / F
f.	Gathered equipment and washed hands.			
g.	Allowed client opportunity to manipulate inhaler. Explained and demonstrated how canister fits into inhaler.	P / F	P / F	P / F
h.	Explained what metered dose is and warned patient about overuse of inhaler.	P / F	P / F	P / F
i.	Explained steps for administering inhaled dose of medication. (1) Removed mouthpiece cover from inhaler. (2) Shook inhaler well. (3) Had client take a deep breathe and exhale. (4) Instructed patient to position inhaler.	P / F	P / F	P / F
j.	With inhaler in proper position, had client hold inhaler with thumb at mouthpiece and index finger and middle finger at the top.	P / F	P / F	P / F
k.	Instructed client to tilt head back slightly, inhale slowly and deeply through mouth, and depressed medication canister fully.	P / F	P / F	P / F
l.	Had patient hold breath for approximately 10 seconds.	P / F	P / F	P / F
m.	Had patient exhale through pursed lips.	P / F	P / F	P / F
n.	Assessed patient's respirations.	P / F	P / F	P / F
o.	Documented procedure.	P / F	P / F	P / F

Instructor Comments:

Wall Mount O2

Soldiers Name: _____ SSN: _____ CO: _____ TM: _____
Start: _____ Stop: _____ Initial Evaluator: _____
Start: _____ Stop: _____ Retest Evaluator: _____
Start: _____ Stop: _____ Final Evaluator: _____

		1st	2nd	3rd
a.	Verified MD/PA orders.	P / F	P / F	P / F
b.	Gathered equipment.	P / F	P / F	P / F
c.	Explained procedure to the patient.	P / F	P / F	P / F
d.	Positioned patient.	P / F	P / F	P / F
e.	Assess patient's airway. (1) Considered laboratory reports of arterial blood gas levels. (2) Suctioned any secretions obstructing the airway (3) Reassessed lung sounds.	P / F	P / F	P / F
f.	Filled humidifier container to designated level.			
g.	Attached flowmeter to humidifier and inserted in proper source.	P / F	P / F	P / F
h.	Administered oxygen via nasal cannula. (1) Attached nasal cannula to oxygen tubing. (2) Attached to flowmeter. (3) Placed prongs in cup of water. Adjusted flow meter to 6 to 10 L to flush tubing and prongs with oxygen. Once water, bubbles, removed and wiped off water. (4) Adjusted flow rate to prescribed amount. (5) Placed nasal prong into each naris of patient. Adjusted liter flow per order. (6) Adjusted straps of cannula over the ears and tighten under the chin. (7) Placed padding between strap and ear.	P / F	P / F	P / F
i.	Administered oxygen via face mask. (1) Adjusted flow rate of oxygen per order. (2) Allowed patient to hold mask and placed hand over patient's hand. (3) Placed mask over bridge of nose, then covered mouth. (4) Adjusted straps around patient's head and over ears. (5) Placed cotton ball or gauze over ears under elastic straps. (6) Observed reservoir bag. Ensure expanding and collapsing with patient's breath.	P / F	P / F	P / F
j.	Maintained regular assessment. (1) Maintained solution in humidifier. (2) Cleaned and dried nares/face as indicated.	P / F	P / F	P / F
k.	Documented procedure.	P / F	P / F	P / F

Instructor Comments:

Wall Mount Suction

Soldiers Name: _____ SSN: _____ CO: _____ TM: _____
Start: _____ Stop: _____ Initial Evaluator: _____
Start: _____ Stop: _____ Retest Evaluator: _____
Start: _____ Stop: _____ Final Evaluator: _____

		1st	2nd	3rd
a.	Verified MD/PA orders.	P / F	P / F	P / F
b.	Explained procedure to the patient.	P / F	P / F	P / F
c.	Gathered necessary equipment	P / F	P / F	P / F
d.	Donned gloves and used mask or face shield.	P / F	P / F	P / F
e.	Opened suction kit/catheter using aseptic technique.			
f.	Filled basin with approximately 100cc of Normal Saline.	P / F	P / F	P / F
g.	Connected one end of connecting tubing to suction machine. (1) Checked to ensure equipment if functioning by suctioning a small amount of water from basin.	P / F	P / F	P / F
h.	Turned on suction device. Set regulator to 80-120mm HG.	P / F	P / F	P / F

Oropharyngeal suctioning

		1st	2nd	3rd
a.	Attached suction catheter to connecting tubing.	P / F	P / F	P / F
b.	Removed oxygen mask. If nasal cannula is used, left in place.	P / F	P / F	P / F
c.	Positioned patient.	P / F	P / F	P / F
d.	Inserted catheter into patient's mouth.	P / F	P / F	P / F
e.	With suction applied, moved catheter around mouth.	P / F	P / F	P / F
f.	Encouraged patient to cough.	P / F	P / F	P / F
g.	Repeated suctioning as needed.	P / F	P / F	P / F
h.	Replaced oxygen mask if removed.	P / F	P / F	P / F
i.	Suctioned water from basin through catheter until the catheter is cleared of secretions.	P / F	P / F	P / F
j.	Placed catheter in clean, dry area.	P / F	P / F	P / F
k.	Turn off suction device.	P / F	P / F	P / F
l.	Disposed of water and cleaned basin.	P / F	P / F	P / F
m.	Removed gloves and washed hands.	P / F	P / F	P / F
n.	Documented procedure.	P / F	P / F	P / F

Nasotracheal suctioning

a.	Attached nonsterile suction tubing to sterile catheter.	P / F	P / F	P / F
b.	Secured catheter to tubing aseptically.	P / F	P / F	P / F
c.	Coated distal 2-3 inches of catheter with water-soluble lubricant.	P / F	P / F	P / F
d.	Removed oxygen delivery device.	P / F	P / F	P / F
e.	Without applying suction, used dominant thumb and forefinger to gently insert sterile catheter into either naris. Inserted during inhalation with slight downward slant.	P / F	P / F	P / F
f.	Inserted catheter approximately 16-20 cm or distance from patient's nose to base of the earlobe.	P / F	P / F	P / F
g.	Applied intermittent suction by placing and releasing nondominant thumb over vent of catheter.	P / F	P / F	P / F
h.	Assess the need to repeat suctioning procedure. (1) Allowed adequate time between suction passes for ventilation and oxygenation. (2) Asked patient to breathe deeply. Encourage coughing. (3) Kept oxygen readily available. (4) Administered oxygen to patient between suctioning attempts.	P / F	P / F	P / F
i.	Performed oral suctioning to clear mouth of secretions.	P / F	P / F	P / F
j.	Rinsed catheter and connection tubing.	P / F	P / F	P / F
k.	Disposed of equipment.	P / F	P / F	P / F
l.	Turned off suctioning device.	P / F	P / F	P / F
m.	Removed gloves and washed hands.	P / F	P / F	P / F
n.	Documented procedure.	P / F	P / F	P / F

Instructor Comments: